The Angiology Bible

Other World Scientific Titles by the Author

Complementary, Alternative Methods and Supplementary Medicine
by G Belcaro
ISBN: 978-1-78634-566-0

Noninvasive Investigations in Vascular Disease
by G Belcaro and A N Nicolaides
ISBN: 978-1-86094-213-6

Once We Were Hunters: A Study of the Evolution of Vascular Disease
by G Belcaro
ISBN: 978-1-86094-262-4 (pbk)

Pharma-Standard Supplements: Clinical Use
by G Belcaro
ISBN: 978-1-78326-933-4
ISBN: 978-1-78326-934-1 (pbk)

The Venous Clinic: Diagnosis, Prevention, Investigations,
Conservative and Medical Treatment, Sclerotherapy and Surgery
by G Belcaro, A N Nicolaides and G Stansby
ISBN: 978-1-86094-051-4

The · Angiology Bible

Giovanni Vincent Belcaro

Irvine³ Vascular Lab, Ch-Pe University, Italy

Supervised by Dr. Maria Rosaria Cesarone

World Scientific

NEW JERSEY · LONDON · SINGAPORE · BEIJING · SHANGHAI · HONG KONG · TAIPEI · CHENNAI · TOKYO

Published by

World Scientific Publishing Europe Ltd.

57 Shelton Street, Covent Garden, London WC2H 9HE

Head office: 5 Toh Tuck Link, Singapore 596224

USA office: 27 Warren Street, Suite 401-402, Hackensack, NJ 07601

Library of Congress Cataloging-in-Publication Data

Names: Belcaro, Giovanni Vincent, author.

Title: The angiology bible / by Giovanni Vincent Belcaro
    (Irvine³ Vascular Lab, Ch-Pe University, Italy).

Description: New Jersey : World Scientific, 2018. | Includes bibliographical references.

Identifiers: LCCN 2018020240 | ISBN 9781786345691 (hc : alk. paper)

Subjects: | MESH: Cardiovascular System | Cardiovascular Diseases

Classification: LCC RC667 | NLM WG 100 | DDC 616.1--dc23

LC record available at https://lccn.loc.gov/2018020240

British Library Cataloguing-in-Publication Data

A catalogue record for this book is available from the British Library.

For any available supplementary material, please visit
https://www.worldscientific.com/worldscibooks/10.1142/Q0169#t=suppl

Desk Editors: Anthony Alexander/Jennifer Brough/Shi Ying Koe

Typeset by Stallion Press
Email: enquiries@stallionpress.com

Preface

This book is a 360° view of vascular pathologies and an introduction to the complexity of the most important field in medicine, with topics including cardiovascular disease, atherosclerosis, venous diseases, investigations, population sciences, prevention and the indication of a specialization field. It offers a broad introduction to angiology and vascular diseases, surgery and medicine, in an easy-to-read format with case studies separated under key areas. The scope includes many different aspects at an introductory level under a single observational point, bringing unity and homogeneity in the otherwise disjointed field of circulation sciences.

Following are some starting points for consideration:

Angiology

Originally, angiology was considered a pure medical specialty. Not anymore. As a specialty dealing with medical aspects of vascular diseases, "angiology" no longer exists in most countries.

Some internists deal very well with vascular problems from a medical point of view, but they cannot be considered "angiologists".

Vascular medicine is the modern evolution of angiology. It is difficult to see any difference.

Possibly, professionals dealing with *vascular medicine* have a deeper interest in research concerning vascular disorders.

Vascular surgery is a defined specialty that in time becomes more technical than clinical, besieged by interventional radiologists for the interventional part and by medical specialists for the noninterventional and preventive aspects.

All original vascular surgeons, who now seem to be near extinction, like Pandas, were general surgeons with specific training, undertaken later in vascular surgical techniques.

Noninvasive investigation is not a specialty but a sector (well defined and highly technological) that may be practiced by several specialists.

It helps when you describe an artery or a vein, having seen one (and preferably many!) in an anatomical or surgical context with all its surroundings and possible interactions with the organs present in the area under exploration. It is a discipline which needs long and intensive training.

Microcirculation testing, effort tests, plethysmography, thermography, etc., are all part of noninvasive investigation.

The use of only ultrasound or Doppler cannot be an inclusive solution for many patients. Physiological tests help to understand physiology and its variations much better.

Circulation sciences

This description includes all the previous branches of vascular medicine and surgery including microcirculation, radiological diagnostic and interventional methods, effort testing and cardiology.

The American Heart Association

The American Heart Association is currently the largest group of practitioners (including physicians involved in basic and clinical research) mastering Circulation Sciences.

Its main meeting (Scientific Sessions) includes all the described aspects of vascular medicine/surgery including the core business of cardiology with very strong sections on pharmacology, thrombosis, imaging, microcirculation, screening and prevention, and the definitive key to our field: "population sciences".

About the Author

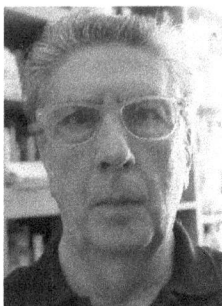

Giovanni V Belcaro is the founder of the Irvine[3] Vascular Lab, Ch-Pe University, Italy and the leader of the San Valentino Vascular Screening Project. He obtained his degree in Medicine and Surgery, then specialized in general surgery and subsequently in thoracic surgery. He obtained a PhD from the University College (St. Mary's Hospital Campus), London working with Mr HHG Eastcott and Prof AN Nicolaides. He has obtained the Imperial College Certificate in Vascular Surgery and Microcirculation (UCL London). He is a fellow of the Royal Society of Medicine, London, UK, a British Council scholar and has worked at Bispebjerg Hospital, Copenhagen. He has authored 30 books and more than 500 scientific articles and original papers. He has attended 300 international meetings. Some of his presentations include those at Westminster and at the European Parliament. He is a member on the editorial board of several international journals. He has worked on and operated different projects in several places including Africa, Philippines, Japan, China, Pakistan and Afghanistan. Among the many research projects he completed, he was the first to implant an artificial Gore-Tex venous valve and use lymphatic transplant. His work on early atherosclerotic plaque evaluation and screening has been a significant progress in the early management of atherosclerosis.

Contents

The Arterial System

1

Arteries

Introduction

Arteries are the anatomical target of the main vascular lesions: all arterial lesions must be considered severe. The major supra-aortic point sites of frequent plaques or stenosis/obstruction and main peripheral points of interest are shown in Figs. 1–3.

The logic of atherosclerosis

Evolution favors the fast accumulators of lipid and proteins. In an original deprivation context (associated to the high level of energy required to find food and preys), fast accumulators have significant nutritional and evolutionary advantages in the pre-reproduction period with faster and better growth and a stronger resistance to deprivation.

After reproduction, with a prolonged life, the fast-effective accumulation becomes a significant negative element creating accumulation of fats and creating plaques which leads to cardiovascular disease. Faster accumulation traits, in association with a sedentary life, also leads to diabetes, weight gain and all other accumulation disorders.

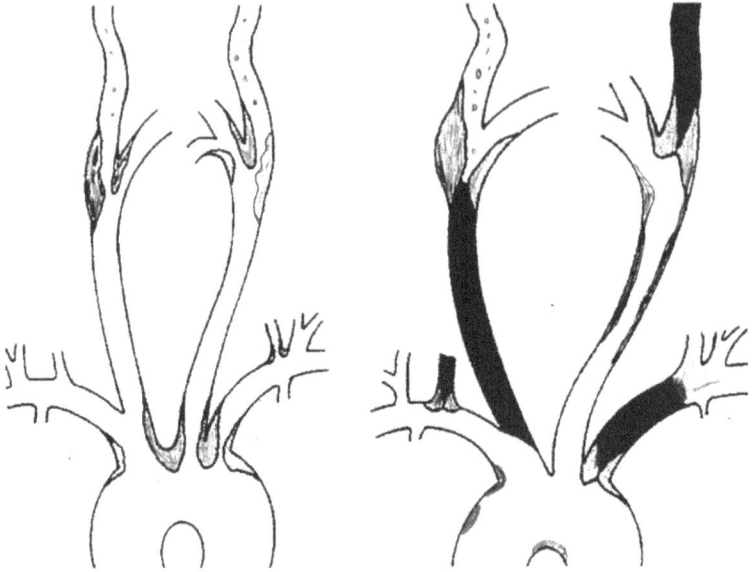

Figure 1.   Most common sovraortic lesions.

Atherosclerosis

Atherosclerosis is generally diffused to the entire arterial system and is very common in humans. It is a condition leading to the formation of arterial thickening, plaques, aneurysms or thrombosis and eventually to occlusion of arteries. Occlusion may be associated with the slow formation or opening of new, more irregular collateral vessels with higher resistance to flow. Some patients with complete occlusion of major arteries may have a sufficient collateral flow preserving function.

When obstruction is rapid (or associated with thrombosis and/or embolization), there is no time for creating a compensatory flow to find an alternative arterial way, and ischemia develops in minutes. The area affected by the ischemia may have a very low tolerance for the reduced or absent perfusion (brain, heart and kidney) that is generally incompatible with regular, basic functions and often with life; some organs may have a

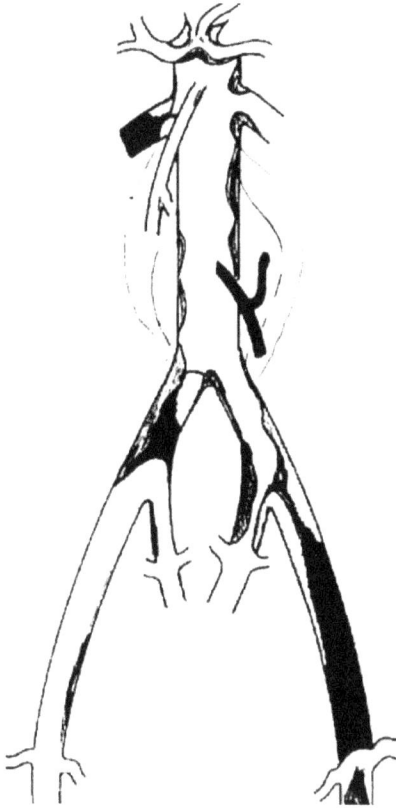

Figure 2.   Most common lesions of the aortic branches.

relatively higher tolerance to ischemia with minimal symptoms or clinical pictures.

Atherosclerosis may kill by obstruction, thrombosis, embolization or aneurysmatic dilatations that may rupture causing sudden and severe bleeding. It is interesting to observe that most of the killers linked to athero-sclerosis can be well documented and even defined in their potential capacity to create dangers, damages or to kill, years before they actually cause a problem. Atherosclerosis is a huge problem, the biggest in industrialized societies, and is largely preventable and can be diagnosed, and it is very often diagnosed or managed in advance.

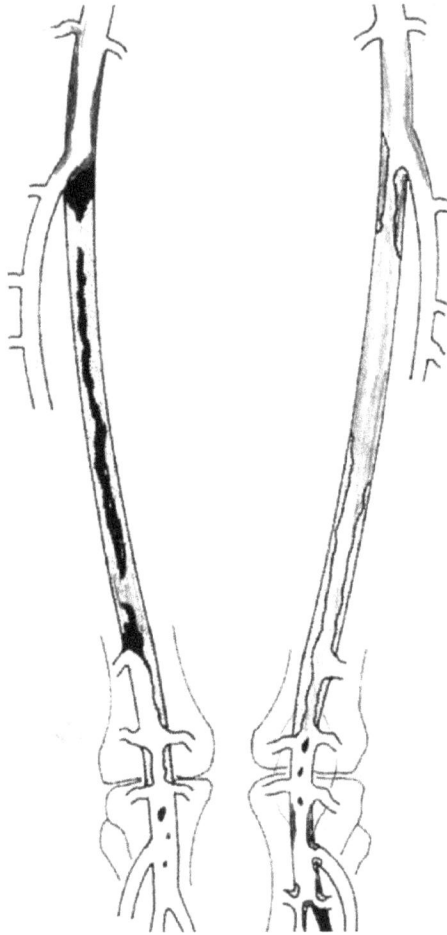

Figure 3.   Common, distal arterial lesions.

Once We Were Hunters (Imperial College Press)[1]

Our evolutionary design was created — for millions of years — in an environment with limited food and a great need of energy to get the food. The combination of a high level of energy and the limited nutritional

---

[1] See *Once We Were Hunters: A Study of the Evolution of Vascular Disease* by G. Belcaro (Imperial College Press).

reward was the push for our evolution. We are still bearing the same evolutionary design in a society with plenty of food and limited need to spend energy to get it. The abundance is only recent (approx. 200 years). The evolutionary design is 5 million years old and still constitutes our basic structure.

The monograph *Once We Were Hunters* investigates this contention in closer detail in the light of what is defined as Darwinian Medicine. Individuals raised in a difficult environment, walking or running all the time to get something to eat or to avoid becoming food, now have plenty of useless food, 10 times more than they need and without walking or running.

Accumulation disorders are the most important problem in our "evolved" society and the fine balance is apparently lost. A "Darwinian" perspective may help to plan early management of atherosclerosis. In the book, one of the points that are discussed is the high incidence of hypertension in the "afro-derived" population in North America. Hypertension is a protective, life-saving factor in scarcity of water. It protects individuals from the effects of dehydration by increasing pressure and perfusion in vital organs. Slaves kept on ships for months in their dramatic voyage from Africa to America suffered often from dehydration. Many died.

Those with higher blood pressure survived and transmitted the pressure trait that was reinforced by the following genetic interactions of individuals with higher levels of pressure. The conditions of the slaves in many plantations actually expanded the value of high pressure and accumulation traits in a general situation of deprivation, dehydration, and food scarcity or irregularities.

The Darwinian view offers an explanation and two solutions for atherosclerosis:

— more exercise
— less food (particularly very caloric elements) and salt (NaCl).

Clinical tips

Noninvasive investigations (e.g., by ultrasound) can detect almost all arterial aneurysms years before they may start to cause serious problems, arterial thickening, or plaques (even defining their potential risk of embolism, thrombosing, or growing faster).

Population screening and population sciences are the key to controlling atherosclerosis but at the moment all the emphasis is generally on medical treatments (drugs) and invasive methods as they lead to significantly higher compensation. Prevention and screening have no sponsors other than government departments who do at least pay lip service to the concepts of prevention and screening. Also, national health systems — at the moment — are just able to cope with sick people (and not all of them in most countries) and do not have time or resources to invest in the healthy population.

Peripheral arterial insufficiency

Human legs and their arteries are bigger, longer and more exposed to arterial blocks than the arteries of the upper limbs. Also, leg arteries have the ability to create collateral circulation, particularly if a block is slow, progressive.

The number and combination of obstructions and their localizations create most symptoms. Diabetic microangiopathy (usually associated with neuropathy) adds other problems by blocking or altering in their functions (including vasodilating or vasoconstricting capacity), the smaller precapillary and capillary arteries, and the distal circulation, including all the microcirculation (that includes all systems of arterial capillaries, microveins and lymphatics).

Both flow in the arteries and perfusion in the capillary bed may become seriously impaired and critically altered. The emphasis — in the recent past — on the measurement of an Ankle Brachial Index (ABI) is now considered obsolete. Subjects with a low ABI are very advanced. Calcification in the arteries may alter the reading.

The visualization of plaques in the arteries — and the quantification of the level of atherosclerosis — with ultrasound can be made 20 or 10 years before there is a difference in pressure between legs and arms that is usually prodromic of severe clinical conditions. Signs/symptoms are not closely linked to ABI but are parallel to the absolute pressure at the level of the tibial arteries.

With a Doppler tibial pressure >80 mmHg, patients may claudicate; with tibial pressures <40 mmHg, most patients tend to have rest or night pain; with less than 25–30 mmHg of pressure, critical ischemia is generally present and in time may evolve into necrosis-gangrene or impending necrosis. With the appropriate combined medical and surgical management, almost no major amputation is now needed and most (97%) of severely ischemic limbs can be saved.

The division of subjects into groups based upon intermittent (better defined as *vascular*) claudication, rest pain, and ischemia-critical limbs is considered purely scholastic/academic. Often in clinical practice there is no progression from one stage to another. Subjects arrive to observation with claudication and have the same problems almost forever (which they have managed to fit within the needs of their life). Progression to the other stages — particularly with management — is now relatively uncommon. Claudicants should be tested with an effort test (preferably on a treadmill or a bike). Care should be taken to avoid stressing the coronary circulation too much.

We have to assume that any patient with vascular claudication and peripheral vascular problems also has a significant degree of coronary problems. We can test the total walking distance, the distance the patient can walk before pain occurs or we can use a faster, easier test (3 min on a treadmill at 3 km/h with 3% inclination). If the subject can perform this test without problems, the impact of the claudication on lifestyle is clini- cally limited. A decrease in heart rate or arterial pressure during the effort test may be a serious indication of coronary problems. The test should be stopped and the cardiologists should take over.

A number of patients with vascular claudication have problems of cardiac output. Improving left ventricular function may increase walking and exercise capacity. Possibly 40% of patients with vascular claudication have other problems (hip, neural compression, disk extrusions, etc.) that require a full clinical contextualization. Too often, the attention (not only in vascular medicine/surgery) is purely technical, only for the limb, one limb or part of it, the rest of the body being left in the dark, out of context. But *the practice of medicine always requires context*: excessive focusing is a wrong technical effort, and can be very misleading. The type of pain of claudicants is variable in localization, timing and consistence; it can be acute, cramping, localized or diffuse.

The distance is expressed in meters (without or with pain). Measuring claudication in city blocks is pointless and does not mean anything in an international context. Some towns do not have blocks in the American style, whereas the meter is the universal measure of distance. Leaving Mr. Leriche to rest in his grave, the complete block of the proximal, iliac arteries may cause significant problems, including erectile dysfunction. By the way, during Vichy, Leriche was appointed the director of the National Medical Board (Ordre des Médecins) created by Pétain and persecuted Jewish physicians.

Generally, the evolution of claudication may be slow and controllable in most patients. The social aspects for vascular claudicants are important, even essential: for example, if you are a policeman or a postman and cannot walk 50 m for a vascular claudication, you may need an aggressive program as it will impact upon your working life. If you are 85 and walk the same distance, the management program may be more conservative and will include your independence to go shopping or perform your most important daily tasks.

Differential diagnosis with arthrosis or bone/joint problems and neuro/spinal compression are common and relatively easy (in these conditions, tibial pressures are normal). Problems may however be concomitant. Coarctation of the aorta, compartment syndromes, masses compressing muscle nerves and arteries (including a possible, rare popliteal entrapment) should be excluded (ultrasound is usually the key evaluation). Neuromuscular compressions tend to be persistent even at rest, in some positions, and not linked to exercise. An exercise test is the diagnostic key particularly in claudicants.

Critical limb ischemia

Critical limb ischemia requires immediate diagnosis and management. With less than 40 mmHg of pressure at the tibial arteries, patients tend to have rest pain; with lower Doppler pressure at the tibial arteries (often the pressure is not measurable), continuous pain and initial ischemia develop. Exact pressure levels can be measured by strain-gauge plethysmography — or laser Doppler flowmetry — particularly when the pressure is very low, flow is slow, and the Doppler signal is not good.

In ischemic conditions, any minimal trauma can cause a skin lesion that does not heal. The burning pain of ischemia is difficult to manage and requires opiates. True ischemia is as distal as anatomy allows (toes). A distal intact foot with an ulceration at the heel needs local evaluation and these lesions are generally a consequence of trauma or compression (e.g., wrong shoes) in ischemic areas.

Rest pain may improve by standing, lowering the limb or walking, but this is only a temporary effect. The ischemic limb may have swelling as it is not used and in some patients, a thrombosis in an ischemic limb — with slow flow — can be the final event leading to more massive ischemia. Neuropathic pain and ischemic pain are differentiated clinically and by the evaluation of the distal perfusion/pressure. Usually, effort tests are not possible in these conditions.

Ulcerations/gangrene or nonhealing ischemic lesions (particularly distal lesions) can be very painful and conditioning the life of the patients.

Healing with ischemic conditions and tibial pressures <30 mmHg simply does not happen unless more perfusion is obtained with medical or interventional methods. Amputation is the last, hopeless solution. Always a defeat. Managing ischemia, infection and pain may allow patients to save a foot for many years. The loss of a foot or a limb in older patients is a devastating event and often a prosthesis is not the possible solution as in younger healthier subjects. The loss of a limb is a serious handicap not only for the patient but also for the family around him. It should be avoided as much as possible.

Main signs/symptoms

Feeling the arteries and peripheral pulses, bruits and looking at the pallor of the limbs, muscle atrophy and a loss of skin annexes — as other signs — is just a basic, initial evaluation. Response to exercise is the most important factor to measure.

A small pocket Doppler should be now in the office of any GP, just like a stethoscope. It is easy to use and can give important information in seconds, separating vascular from nonvascular patients, detecting a real perfusional problem, giving a quantitative value to any observation. Measuring Doppler (tibial) pressure is the next step and it can be done in minutes. Palpating the arteries or feeling pulses may be misleading in large or overweight patients.

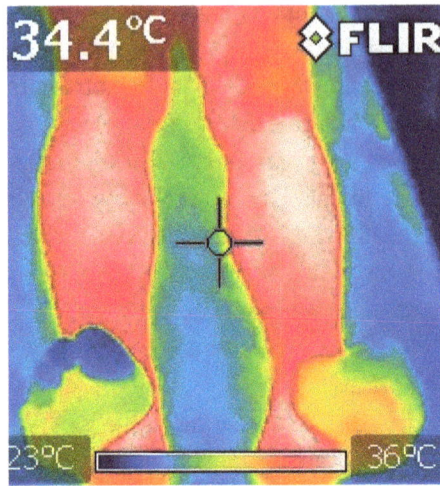

Figure 4.   Thermographic evaluation of an outpatient panoramically showing hypoperfused areas and thermographic asymmetries in seconds. Perfusional asymmetry at the distal right foot.

A thermographic evaluation (Fig. 4) panoramically shows hypoperfused areas and thermographic asymmetries in seconds, and it allows the screening of normal from abnormal, also giving a fast quantitative and anatomical value to perfusional problems. Ultrafast thermography now is mobile, fast, independent from environmental temperature and may show easily perfusional deficits in seconds.

An exercise test is the definitive key, noninvasive test for the patients that *are* able to take it (claudicants and most subjects with rest pain can tolerate the test). The total walking distance — the most important diagnostic-prognostic number — can be measured by defining the distance the patients can walk without pain or the total, tolerated distance. Short-range claudication (<80 m) may cause a disappearance or peripheral pulses for some time. The time needed to regain pulses can also be considered.

Generally, ABI is not useful. It is only a very late screening method. The walking distance is more than enough for defining a diagnosis and can be used as a target for the evaluations of the progression with management. When the pain is not vascular, there is no drop in peripheral pressure with the exercise test and exercise may actually improve pain.

Case 1. Hypoperfusion of all toes and distal feet. Symptoms: rest pain, severe claudication, distal tibial arteries not detectable. Treatment with prostaglandin E1 (PGE1) infusions (60 μg/d in 100 mL in 30 min). Improvement in 3D.

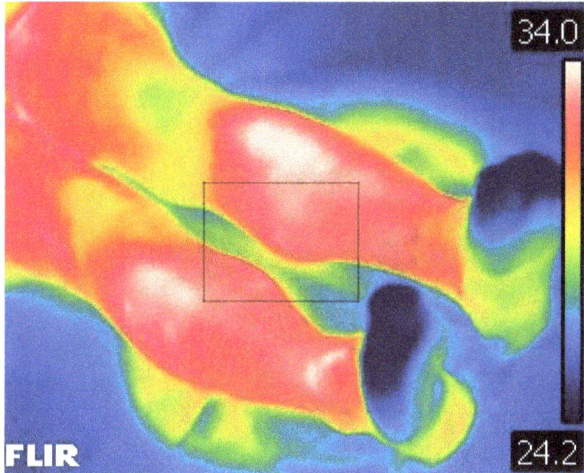

Case 2. Altered distal perfusion: toes and fingers. Ischemic external/anterior foot. Severe pain at rest. Good perfusion of foot. Treatment with PGE1. Improvement; no need for amputation.

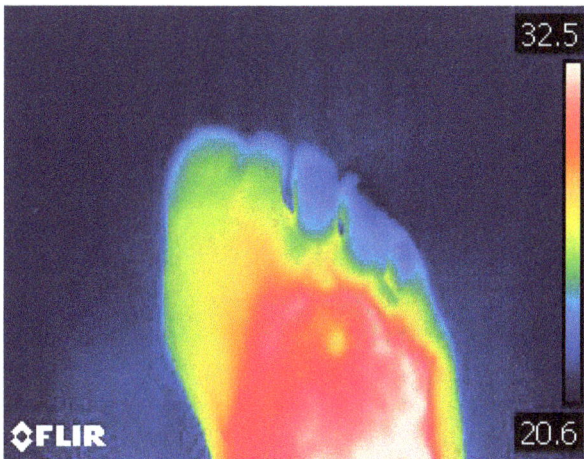

Case 3. (a) Ischemia and pain of third and fourth fingers in subject (fisherman) working with ice. Management: prevention and protection from cold and exposure with specific thermic gloves. Improvement in days; no need for medical treatment. (b) Thermic glove for prevention and protection from cold and exposure.

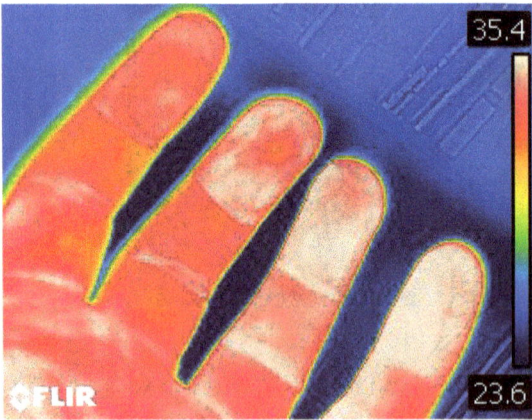
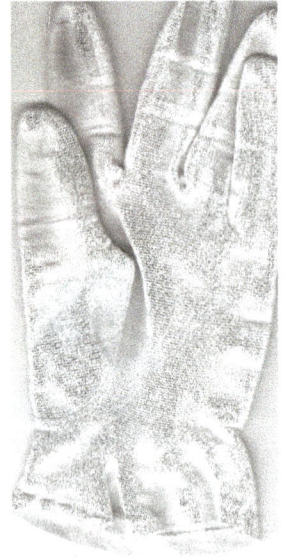

(a)   (b)

2

Noninvasive Investigations

Introduction

Starting with a simple pocket Doppler, ultrasound tests are usually diagnostic. Color duplex is needed to evaluate plaques, the localization of the most effected segment, to define the characteristics of the lesions and to visualize flow and slow flow distally to occlusions. The different ultrasound tests give most of the needed anatomical data; duplex evaluations include the aorta, the iliac arteries and all the peripheral vessels.

The idea that color duplex ultrasound is "operator dependent" is faulty. Anything in medicine depends on the experience and commitment of the operators. Also, some duplex scanners are very essential and cost <$20,000; other more complex machines cost >$100,000 and produce different results in more detail, produce better imaging, show flow characteristics and offer a diagnostic speed.

Good scanners and good doctors get the best results. But if you buy a Steinway, you do not automatically become Rachmaninoff. To become skillful requires good training and constant practice and clinical background. Noninvasive investigations require years of clinical practice and this is just not standardized at the moment. The clinical understanding of any disease is the best basis for a successful, satisfactory test. For most subjects with claudication, however, noninvasive tests are more than adequate to help diagnose their problems and commence effective treatment as soon as possible.

Invasive tests

Angiography, which includes different types and modalities of invasive vascular tests (usually CT angio or CTA), is designed to show the lumen of the arteries and the level of stenosis. The use of contrast may be nephrotoxic, cause allergy and may cause several problems. CTA is therefore used only when

(a) noninvasive tests are inconclusive or disappointing and cannot produce a good documentation for a valid diagnosis (<10% of cases),
(b) an interventional action is already planned (usually for advanced patients with rest pain or ischemia).

Distal, smaller arteries are difficult to see with angiography and images may be obstructed by calcifications. Selective angiography can get better results in these cases. MR angiography (MRA) may give similar images with visualization of distant vessels. Angiography shows details of the affected vessel and the distal run-off and collaterals. It is usually used only in subjects in need of interventional procedures (mainly surgery). It is considered the morphological gold standard.

However, injection of contrast at higher-than-physiological pressure may show vessels that are not perfused at normal (e.g., <60 mmHg) pressure in the limb with vascular obstruction. Even an injection by hand can easily reach a pressure of >300 mmHg. At that pressure you may see something that it is not there in adapted-physiological and perfusional conditions in a system accustomed to work at an average pressure <80–50 mmHg.

Contrast agents may cause reactions and contrast-induced renal failure is a reality. Therefore, the use of angiography should be selective and associated with proper management (hydration, limited infusion of contrast). Angiography is morphology: the symptoms are caused by physiology (variation in pressure) not always parallel to morphology. Angiography and CT angio should not be routinely used for claudicants who may be usually managed with noninterventional therapeutic plans.

When more than one determinant stenosis is present, it would be useful to measure pressure before and after (proximally and distally) each occlusion. Treatment may be selectively dedicated to the most significant occlusion: for example, a femoral occlusion decreases pressure from 130 to 80 mmHg; a popliteal stenosis/obstruction decreases pressure to some 30 mmHg). The final tibial pressure is around 50 mmHg. The correction of the femoral stenosis should bring the tibial pressure from 30 to some 110 mmHg. There is no need to correct the popliteal problem as most patients with this level of tibial pressure become asymptomatic.

The association of physiological measurements with very selective angiography — in critically ischemic limbs — may offer the best results with minimal effort. As indicated, the injection of contrast during angiography may show vessels that are not there at the physiological pressure of the claudicant. Results of revascularization into "ghost" vessels may be very disappointing. Even a satisfactory postrevascularization angiogram, if the pressure of infusion of contrast is high, may show an effective revascularization, with visible run-off that would not be visible at lower levels of pressure.

Management

Peripheral vascular disease is not only a severe problem but also a very severe marker of advanced atherosclerosis. Patients tend to die from strokes or myocardial infarction (MI); now they do not generally die from peripheral vascular disease. Renal failure is a very bad prognostic factor as these patients tend to die within 2–3 years. Smoking as a factor also increases the risk of lung tumors in most patients.

Diabetes, if not controlled, tends to lower life expectancy and to cause several other problems from local, systemic and eye/retinal problems, etc. Well-controlled diabetes, even advanced, may have a less severe effect on mortality times and on complications.

Noninterventional, conservative management: diet, aggressive reduction of risk factors (smoking, obesity, a sedentary life, hypertension, etc.) should be considered and managed appropriately. Now every patient seen by a vascular specialist is managed with antihypertensives, lipid-lowering agents, antiplatelet agents and very often diet, although lifestyle — not having sponsorships — is often left untouched. The management of risk factors requires discipline and makes even more sense in younger subjects. In older subjects, too much pharmacotherapy may cause further problems, eventually creating more complications than it was originally intended to prevent.

Statins may cause significant problems (muscular and myocardial dysfunctions, hepatic and renal problems) and alternative managements (diet and fish oil for instance or supplementation with CoQ10) might be considered as a way of lessening the statin load.

For vascular patients, there is always an individual management and a delicate balance. It is not possible to give everybody the same products at the same quantities. Hypertriglyceridemia may be managed with other drugs but is ultimately a matter of diet modification. The same can be said for most diabetic patients.

Often patients use drugs to control the condition, but few make more than a little effort to control their diet and heighten their levels of exercise. Glycosylated hemoglobin >7% can be a significant factor in increasing the rate of progression of vascular disease and the rate of complications. It is often a significant clinical measure of the attention of the patients.

Exercise and rehabilitation

Management with simple daily walks and regular exercise may be very effective for most claudicants. Supervision is rarely needed unless patients have special problems. A family tutor or a friend — identified within the patient's circle — may be briefed to help.

Subjects with claudication tend to spontaneously restrict their walking. The more frequent use of cars limits the perception of claudication in many patients. Asking or gently forcing them to walk and exercise more frequently or longer may increase even 2–3 times the walking distance, thereby improving muscular performance and resistance. The improvement in exercise level may also have important effects on risk factor management (e.g., hypertension, diabetes and lipids). Almost all claudicants can be therefore managed with exercise and control of risk factors.

The use of prostaglandins

Prostaglandins (in particular PGE1) are the drugs of choice for peripheral vascular disease. The use of prostaglandin PGE1 is safe, well tolerated and relatively cheap. It can easily double the walking distance (e.g., even with a weekly infusion of 60–80 mg) in 30 min, in an outpatient setting. After 4 weeks, most patients double, at least, their walking distance. Perfusion also improves at renal, cardiac and cerebral levels and at the foot level.

PGE1 is the safest and best tolerated among prostaglandins. However, as many other products not produced in the USA, it is not frequently used in the USA, the leading market; actually, it is generally ignored, not even mentioned in most medical texts and articles as the treatment of choice for peripheral vascular disease. At the moment, it is the main core drug for the management of claudicants and critical limb ischemia (both subjects with rest pain and necrosis have significant benefits) with several personalized therapeutic plans.

PGE1 also increases survival rate in these patients decreasing myocardial event and strokes and improving kidney perfusion and functions. PGE1 infusions do not compete with surgery or other noninterventional or interventional methods and can be integrated into a comprehensive global management of any ischemic condition.

Antiplatelet agents

Antiplatelet agents are not a treatment or the therapy for atherosclerosis; they are used for an (arterial) antithrombotic prophylaxis. Massive studies have shown a number of activities of most antiplatelet agents including increase in claudication distances (but it is a very limited increase).

Most studies including more than 20,000 patients have shown benefits as antiplatelet agents appear to decrease the incidence of events (strokes, transient ischemic attacks (TIAs) and myocardial infarctions). Actually, if you need a study with 20,000 subjects to show something, the benefit of the drug could be marginal. Very big studies are good to evaluate safety but not necessarily good to show efficacy. In pneumonia, you need five patients to show the effects of antibiotics.

The side effects and costs of aspirin and other antiplatelet agents are often important; side effects may be severe and even deadly. Retinal hemorrhage, brain bleeding, gastric complications should be considered. Around 25% of patients cannot use aspirin; in some subjects, aspirin appears to be ineffective (possibly 7%) and side effects including microbleeding may be seen, in time, in another percentage of patients.

There is not a single study that shows that atherosclerotic plaques are reduced in size or that plaques progression becomes slower with anti-platelet agents. Therefore, antiplatelet agents are an antithrombotic prophylaxis, possibly very useful to prevent a number of cases of embolization but at significant cost. It is possibly wrong to give every patient antiplatelet agents all the time, and independent, selective studies (not meta-analysis) are needed.

Case 1. Subjects working in a supermarket with frozen food. Severe symmetrical ischemia involving all fingers. Management: protection and PGE1 infusion (40 μg in infusions, twice a week for 2 months. Improvement in days.

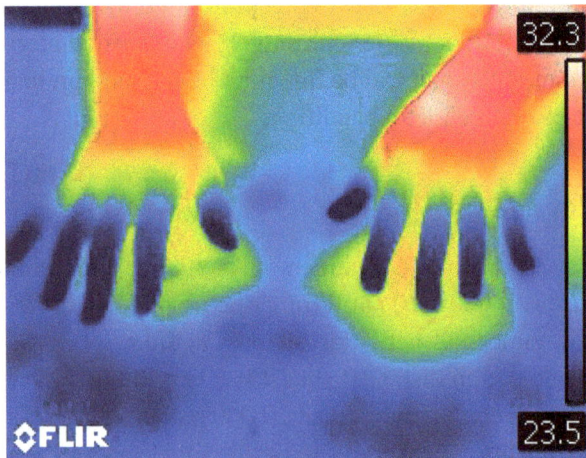

3

Interventional Treatments

Introduction

Interventional treatments are generally indicated in patients with rest pain or ischemia/gangrene. Careful blending of medical and surgical methods is essential. General conditions, as for any type of surgery, may indicate the best interventional possibility for most patients.

Endovascular procedures

Endovascular procedures treat the arterial segments from inside the arteries. A percutaneous access into the arterial system (e.g., the common femoral artery) allows the passage of a catheter under fluoroscopy. When the target segment of the lesion is reached, angioplasty may dilate the arterial lumen and stents can be placed to keep the lumen at the obtained size and with a regular flow.

Most procedures are minimally invasive and have many advantages compared with open surgery. Minimally invasive procedures — also in association with medical treatment (PGE1) — can be an important choice in higher risk individuals with critical limb ischemia which is not manageable with medical treatments alone.

Long-term patency and efficiency of endovascular methods are difficult to predict as there are many procedures, stents, combination of conditions including the progress in atherosclerosis in single individuals. Generally, most procedures are effective, relatively safe and may last.

Stenting

From the aorta to the popliteal, most arterial arteries can be stented. Below-knee arteries can be accessed and treated with smaller catheters. Percutaneous mechanical or laser-based atherectomy can be also associated with the angioplasty.

Usually, short vascular lesions may be better treated with angioplasty. The stenotic segment is expanded and flow is regained; stents improve and keep the luminal enlargement and protect against restenosis. Longer stents (stent grafts) may be used in the case of suspected ruptures during angioplasty and for longer lesions. Drug-eluting stents improve patency. However, larger arteries and smaller/shorter lesions have the best outcome. The outcome is however a balance between treatment methods, atherosclerosis progression, patient's behavior and the associated medical treatment.

Distal arterial segments and complex, multiple lesions may have a less satisfactory outcome. However, even an 80% patency at 1 year may be a positive perfusional shock for the patient and the limb, improving signs/symptoms, restoring mobility in most cases, and giving an opportunity to stimulate a larger, new collateral circulation.

Repeated procedures (with angioplasty, stenting) tend to have less and less efficacy and should be considered on an individual basis. The costs of minimally interventional procedures are high and should be considered.

Surgical reconstruction

Aorto-iliac reconstruction with open surgery could be indicated in patients with a longer life expectancy, severe and multiple-segments disease not easily treatable with endovascular procedures. Flow is restored to the femoral arteries (superficial femoral artery, if patent, or to the profunda femoris artery). If peripheral runoff is adequate, the patency of the reconstruction tends to be good at 5 years (around 80%). In this context, the profunda femoris artery can be enlarged, treated with endarterectomy and its flow improved. This artery supplies a large quantity of blood to muscles, and it is very useful to improve the collateral circulation.

As in any major surgery, operative risks and all possible complications should be considered (anastomotic aneurysms, renal failure, erectile dysfunction). In high-risk subjects, alternative procedures can be considered (e.g., iliofemoral bypass). Extra-anatomic procedures (e.g., axillofemoral grafts) tend to be less successful and are becoming less frequent. A short, larger, bypass with a good runoff the is the key to patency in this surgery. Distal (i.e., femoropopliteal) reconstruction is used for limb survival.

Indications are variable and individual and associated with the presence of a viable vessel to revascularize. Small caliber polytetrafluoroethylene (PTFE) grafts can be used but veins — if available — are the best options for these distal bypasses. Tibial or peroneal reconstructions, when possible, are technically difficult and used only for limb survival; veins are the preferred grafts. Complications and limited survival in this type of patients should be considered.

Amputation

Amputation, clearly, is the last option and it becomes compulsory

(a) when pain is untreatable,
(b) when infection and/or gangrene become a life risk for the patient.

Limitation of the need for amputations is possible using intensive PGE1 infusion, with a combination of medical and surgical methods; amputations have been greatly delayed, controlled and reduced recently.

Postamputation prosthesis — Yes or no

The idea that a prosthesis is better than a bad limb is debatable. A prosthesis with its long, re-education process is better in younger, otherwise healthy individuals who are more likely to be adaptable. Older subjects react very badly to an amputation as it is, and often, do not have the muscular power or the motivation/psychological strength to persevere with prostheses. For these patients, amputation is often considered an almost-terminal event that affects not only their body but also all family members.

No Man Is an Island; amputation is not only a personal but also a social loss in our efficientistic society. Patients and their family circles all lose. Patients should, therefore, be carefully counseled and helped. Most patients prefer to live with a chronic lesion in the foot if the pain is controllable (and having to regularly change their dressing) than to lose a limb.

PGE1 infusions and pain management is the real key, and may be very effective in controlling and reducing the need for amputation. All vascular centers should include methods for decreasing the number of amputations required as an annual target.

4

Acute Vascular Occlusions, Thrombosis and Embolization

Introduction

A fast obstruction in the arterial system is a physiologically catastrophic, rapidly progressive event. Symptoms are a combination of flow blockage and often a concomitant, reactive, massive vasoconstriction that may block the possible collateral perfusion.

Embolization or acute thrombosis or a combination of the two conditions is the cause of most acute obstruction (excluding traumatic events). Embolization from the heart (atrial fibrillation, valves, rare tumors) is the most frequent but emboli can be produced by the aorta by complex arterial plaques or aneurysmal sacs. A small number of embolic sources cannot be identified (some 10%). Even venous thrombi can embolize into the arterial system via a patent foramen ovale (PFO) (it is a rare event but less rare than previously believed).

Clinically, embolization and thrombosis may be comparable. An embolus can be immediately followed by a proximal thrombosis progressively extending proximally and blocking collaterals.

Signs/symptoms

Limb pain is the key. The loss of sensation may be a sign of severe neurological ischemia. Muscle tissue can die from ischemia within hours. The limb becomes pallid and hypothermic. Distal pulses are not detectable by Doppler. Diffuse edema may follow in some cases.

Treatment

Anticoagulants block the propagation of the thrombus and give some time for a better evaluation. When possible, arteriography can be performed to study the anatomy of the vessels and plan a revascularization if needed. An almost normal arterial tree may suggest distal embolization (from the heart).

Catheter thrombolysis, percutaneous thrombectomy or open surgical embolectomy must be used according to individual needs. With a Fogarty catheter, the embolus with its thrombotic tail can be extracted in minutes. After hours of occlusion, the adhesion of the thrombus to the wall (and its extension) make embolectomy more complex and less satisfactory.

In acute ischemia, interventional methods may restore flow in minutes. The association of thrombotic agents may improve embolectomy. In less acute cases thrombolytic agents (tissue plasminogen activator) can be infused into the clot. Surgical revascularization may be needed to prevent new clotting at the level of complex plaques. Minor obstructions may positively respond to heparin and PGE1 infusions.

Reperfusion injury

After a persisting (hours) obstruction, myoglobin recirculated from the damaged muscles may reach the kidneys causing renal insufficiency. Hydration and appropriate medical management should avoid this severe complication.

The massive vasodilatation of the ischemic tissue, distal to the obstruction, may produce, when flow is restored, massive edema in the ischemic areas that requires treatment to avoid compartment syndrome and further ischemia.

Intermittent pneumatic compression for arterial assistance

Intermittent pneumatic compression pumps have a long, efficacious history of use for the prevention of deep vein thrombosis, chronic venous insufficiency and lymphatic disorders.

Arterial assist pumps are a very different form of pneumatic compression used for the treatment of peripheral arterial disease. Because the foot and toes are often involved in lower extremity ischemia, arterial assist pumps have limb cuffs that include foot and calf compression bladders. Since they are used in the sitting position with higher internal hydrostatic vascular pressures, they must supply much higher pressures than other pump types; typically, around 120 mmHg or three to four times that of their venous and lymphatic counterparts.

Their primary mechanism of action is based on the high levels of vascular wall shear stress applied to the endothelium from a very rapid application of pressure, taking less than 500 ms to reach peak pressure and holding for a very short time.

In response to shear stress, the endothelium releases various biochemical components including nitric oxide, tissue growth factors and fibrinolytics. Nitric oxide causes immediate vasodilation at the arteriolar level which reduces peripheral resistance and therefore increases blood flow at the tissue level.

Over time, collateral arteries grow; these arteries tend to form a natural bypass around obstructed arteries. This results in a durable improvement when used in intermittent claudication and critical limb ischemia.

Figure 1 shows the acute effect of intermittent pneumatic compression and popliteal artery flow before compression and after compression. Note end-diastolic flow due to reduced peripheral resistance. Long-term effect can be seen on angiography with increase in collateral circulation after 3–4 months of use.

(a)   (b)

(c)   (d)

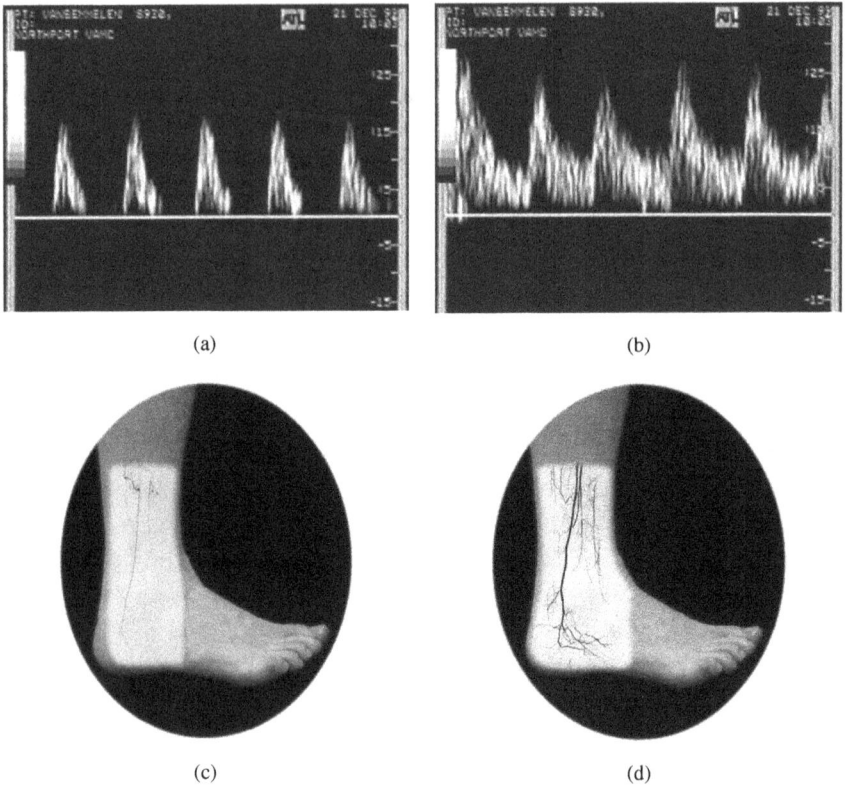

Figure 1.   Acute effect of intermittent pneumatic compression. Severe distal vasoconstriction (no diastolic flow). (a) Popliteal artery flow before compression. (b) Presence of
end-diastolic flow due to reduced peripheral resistance after intermittent pneumatic compression. (c) and (d) Long-term effect. Substantial increase in collateral circulation growth
after 3–4 months of use.

Traumatic arterial occlusion

These lesions may occur acutely, often in association with other bone or
muscular injuries. They must be repaired as soon as possible. Bleeding
may kill in minutes.

There is no time to develop any collateral in most cases. Common
arterial and venous injuries often with nerve involvement as the result of,
e.g., accidents require rapid and complex management. Even a temporary

repair and revascularization may save limbs, thereby allowing other surgical repairs. Repair or reflow of arteries must be done before repairing other injuries. Consider that collateral flow in otherwise healthy individuals may efficiently bypass arterial interruptions that may be well tolerated in time.

5

Small Arteries/Microcirculation

Introduction

Serious distal arterial disease when the occlusion involves the terminal circulation, distal organs and tissues, without the possibility of collateral revascularization (e.g., in toes), may rapidly lead to necrosis. Embolization also produces rapid distal necrosis. To have embolization traveling to the more distal arteries, the proximal arteries should be free from obstruction (as in embolization from the heart in younger subjects). The source of embolization should be aggressively detected to avoid more emboli.

Anticoagulants, acute PGE1 infusions and the interventional method are used to treat the ischemic tissues. The source of embolization may require specific management (valvular replacement, anticoagulants). Multiple microemboli — causing peripheral TIAs — in different areas may be diagnostic of an embolizing source. Sudden discoloration, pain numbness, microinfarctions cause toe or distal foot cyanosis. Cardiac and vascular source, aorta, femoral/aortic plaques should be all considered and if possible treated.

Microembolization

With very small emboli, the aspect of the limb may be normal even with the tibial arteries patent. The aspect of an almost normal foot with good perfusion and localized ischemic area may be typical. Amputation can be avoided in most patients; in some patients, a spontaneous resolution may be observed.

Diabetic vascular disease

Common distal calcified arteries, with asymmetrical perfusional defects are associated with lesions often consequent to minor daily trauma in areas with very limited nutritional perfusion and altered nerve functions.

Necrosis, almost always caused by small trauma, edema (the hallmark of diabetic microangiopathy) and neuropathy, which is often associated, may lead to tissue loss and serious local infections, which may prove difficult to heal.

Small arteries, generally <1 mm in diameter tend to be involved. The combination neuropathy, microangiopathy, edema, anesthesia or altered sensations in various formats make this frequent combination very complex to manage. More proximal arterial problems and even distal tibial arterial lesions tend to be associated as atherosclerosis and diabetes are generally associated.

In diabetics, advanced atherosclerosis tends to progress faster, being more progressive than vascular disease alone. ABI is generally useless when arteries are calcified, as very high pressure may be needed to occlude the tibial arteries. Foot pressure measurements may be difficult. The real perfusional pressure with definition of critical levels of ischemia can be made with strain-gauge plethysmography or laser Doppler flowmetry.

Thermography is a very useful and simple screening method to detect altered distal perfusion (Fig. 1). Management is mainly medical with PGE1. Most distal bypasses are complex, arteries are very small and the grafts have a high rate of failure considering the poor and limited run-off.

Atherosclerotic lesions and microangiopathy have two different, concomitant evolution and expression and usually require parallel managements. Foot care and management is essential (protection of skin and toes, soft shoes, prevention and control of any infection, mirror to see nonvisible spots). Diabetic control is essential but the course of diabetic control on the evolution of microangiopathy is not always parallel. In some patients, microangiopathy can be present on

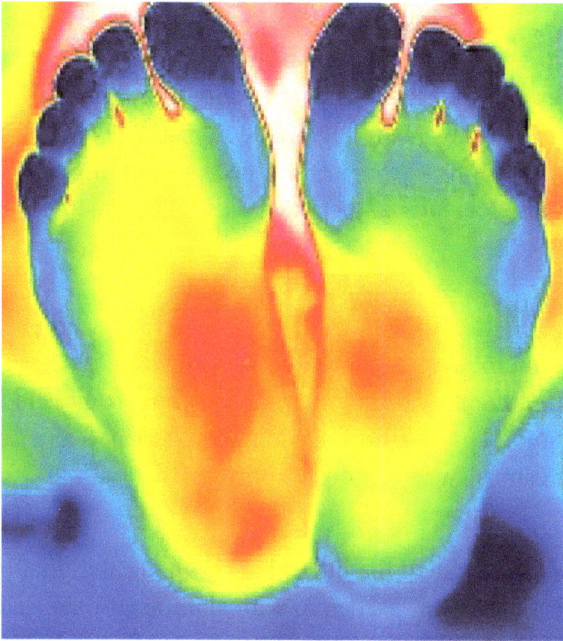

Figure 1. Severe distal hypoperfusion seen by thermography in seconds. The left heel — external side — is also more ischemic than the contralateral area and shows small skin lesions.

prediabetic stages. Dry skin breaks more frequently and easily. Minor breaks do not heal easily without careful management and may lead to larger and deeper lesions.

Differentiating the damages due to microangiopathy, neuropathy and atherosclerosis has a significant clinical value and requires specific managements. Microangiopathy also involves retinal vessels, kidney, brain and coronary vessels and the whole vascular system.

The venoarteriolar response (VAR) — namely, the reflex axon–axon response to standing and increases in pressure at the distal vascular levels, measurable at the distal skin with laser Doppler — is significantly altered; this leads to the formation of edema. The functional alterations of the VAR may be present years before the microcirculation is finally anatomically compromised.

Microcirculation studies are the key to fully understand and follow up microangiopathic changes in diabetic patients. Good, early detection

— defining the patients and limbs at higher risk of microangiopathy — and a specific early management reduces the number of amputations. Stockings prevent edema — when present — in most diabetic patients avoiding progression of microangiopathy. Prostaglandin E1 management with regular infusions may prevent necrosis in higher-risk subjects, improving healing or microangiopathic lesions in most patients.

Other microangiopathies

Several other microangiopathies may be induced by diseases or by pharmacological treatments. The definition and management is individual and, generally all microangiopathies leading to ischemia, decreased perfusion and necrosis respond well to infusions of PGE1.

Case 1. Severe ischemia of the little finger with distal digital ischemia and initial skin lesions. Severe ischemia with significant pain (lady, 40 years, no other significant problems) occurred, in days, after treatment with interferon for a dubious diagnosis of rheumatoid arthritis. Full resolution with four infusions of PGE1 (40 μg/d in 100 mL). No other consequences.

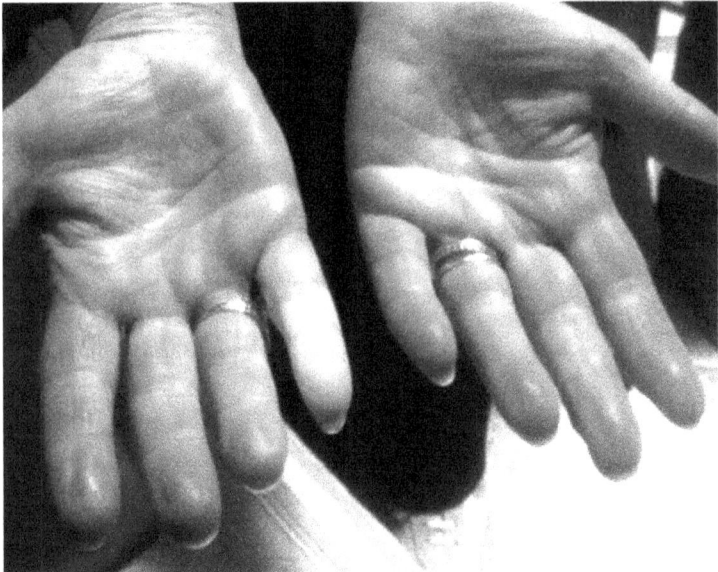

6

Nonathero Vascular Disease

Thromboangiitis obliterans

Thromboangiitis obliterans is now a debatable clinical entity, usually considered to affect young male smokers with a strong inflammatory component. A purely nonatherosclerotic vascular disease is very rare and most management, e.g., adding an anti-inflammatory management — if inflammation is present and significant — may help some patients. Corticosteroids may help some patients. The general management (including an aggressive control of all risk factors) is comparable to the general management for atherosclerosis and diabetic microangiopathy.

Diffuse, repeated "phlebitis" can be a rare observation in some individuals; these symptoms are possibly more frequent in some populations and conditions. The clinical conditions associated to Buerger's disease are observed less frequently now. Some toxic reaction in the patients' history, some aspecific or specific immunological patterns may be found. Antibodies may attack arterial antigens. Buerger's disease affects arteries and veins in the arms and legs. This eventually damages tissues also leading to infections and gangrene. Usually this condition initially appears at the hands and feet and eventually may affect larger sections of the limbs. Subjects diagnosed with this disease have a tobacco dependency. Avoiding tobacco is considered the only way to stop the disease. Painful lesions, amputations may follow in noncompliant patients.

Noninvasive investigations and angiography can be unusual but nonspecific. History and clinical aspects are diagnostic. Sympathectomy now is not used anymore. PGE1 treatment — often in association with heparin — has significant effects of symptoms, particularly on ischemic distal lesions allowing healing in a relatively short time.

Selective antibiotics (or antimycotic treatments) and anti-inflammatory agents may help and corticosteroids may be effectively used in subjects with a higher inflammatory component. Amputations may be needed very early in the evolution of the disease.

However, the combination of PGE and corticosteroids — if erythrocyte sedimentation rate (ESR) is high — and control of possible infections and risk factors may now effectively control this condition and decrease the need for amputations. For some reason, we have not seen any of these patients for many years.

Popliteal entrapment

Popliteal entrapment (PoEn) is considered a rare condition: the popliteal artery passes between two heads of the gastrocnemius muscle. The popliteal artery — in symptomatic patients with PoEn — is medial to both heads causing particularly compression when the knee is extended. The compression, in time, leads to a fibrous thickening of the artery, with dilatations, thrombosis or occlusion. These patients are generally, young subjects, with claudication or pain in some position of the limb; pain due to nerve compression can be present.

Muscular hypertrophy may be also observed. Moving the leg/foot in some specific positions may completely block distal flow and pulses are lost. MRI can be used to see compression (evaluating the limb in different positions) and angio, in the right, occluding position, may show the problem.

Management: There are different solutions with open surgery to correct the compression; some cases may be treated with stents; in some patients, a bypass is needed. In some other earlier cases — when the artery is not damaged — surgery involves the compressing structures (muscles and tendons).

Cystic degeneration

Cystic degeneration of the popliteal artery is a rare disease associated with mucoid cysts developing in the adventitia. Reduced peripheral pulses and a palpable mass are observed in some patients; a circular arterial wall thickening can be seen by ultrasound. The affected arterial segments must be excised and bypassed when possible. Some cases may be possibly treated with endovascular methods now. However, the condition is uncommon and endovascular experience is still limited.

Abdominal aortic coarctation

Rare, congenital processes are associated with this condition, possibly resulting from chronic inflammatory processes such as Kawasaki or Takayasu. Coarctation may be observed in association with distal ischemia related to the degree of the coarctation and its anatomic level that

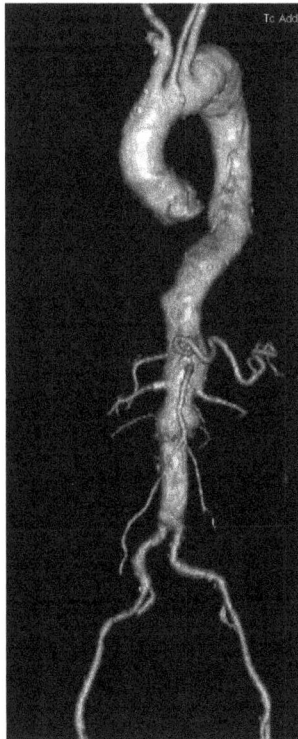

Figure 1.   3D reconstructions from CT or MR scans are possible with specific software (Osirix) and give a complete panoramic image of the aorta that can be rotated and seen under different points of view.

may include mesenteric or kidney ischemia and impotence. Difference in pressure between arms and legs can be initially diagnostic.

Surgical management may now include endovascular procedures and/ or stents when possible (short segment and good arterial walls). In younger subjects, surgery is now very satisfactory: surgery tends to avoid, when possible, the use of artificial prostheses for better long-term results.

When it is present, inflammation should be treated considering ERS and other inflammatory markers. Three-dimensional (3D) reconstructions from CT or MR scans are possible with specific software (e.g., Osirix) and give a complete panoramic image of the aorta that can be rotated and seen under different angles (see Fig. 1).

7

Vasculitis

Introduction

Vasculitis is an inflammatory condition of blood vessels associated to several clinical conditions. Vasculitis can be generalized or localized to one organ or system (e.g., skin, kidney or heart).

What is defined as Primary vasculitis, apparently, is not associated to a specific known cause or etiological agents. Secondary vasculitis may be associated to drugs, toxins, infections, normal or abnormal antigens or associated to other diseases and clinical conditions.

The pathophysiology of most vasculitic diseases (VDs) is difficult to understand but it is often associated to the deposition of some immune complexes in the walls of arteries/veins. Several immune mechanisms may be involved in this process.

Genetic causes may be observed in some conditions; some initial trigger may initiate the immunological process that progressively extends itself in time and to many organs/systems without a self-limiting mechanism. All main types of vessels (arteries, arterioles, capillaries, venules and veins) may be involved.

Arteries and organ damages are generally due to localized arterial necrosis that may cause thrombosis or arterial/flow obstruction. The histological changes observed in most vasculitis are broadly comparable. In most acute histological pictures, polymorphonuclear leukocytes (PMNs) are the predominant inflammatory cells while in chronic clinical evolution, lymphocytes are the most common cells observed in the inflamed tissues.

The localization of the lesion may involve only a segment of some arteries in some cases but in other, the entire artery can be involved. Cellular infiltrations and tissue necrosis and eventually scarring may affect one or more layers of the vessels.

Medial inflammation of muscular arteries, progressively, tends to destroy the internal elastic lamina. Vessel wall inflammation eventually leads to fibrosis and intimal thickening and hypertrophy. Intimal hypertrophy and thickening and associated thrombosis alter and eventually occlude the arterial lumen often leading to tissue ischemia and necrosis.

After the initial vessel lesions when the integrity of the vessel is altered, white cells and fibrin accumulate and leak into the surrounding connective tissue. Specific histologic changes may therefore develop in association with specific clinical pictures (e.g., giant cells and destruction of the internal lamina can be observed in giant cell arteritis).

Classification

Vasculitis-associated disorders (VADs) can be classified (*Merck Manual*, 19th edition, 2011) according to size–depth involvement of the affected vessels. There is an overlap amongst most VADs which contributes to several other diseases. Systemic necrotising vasculitis (SNV) generally involves medium-sized vessels and may produce infarctions in several organs and systems. Vasculitic conditions include the following:

1. Behçet's syndrome
2. Churg–Strauss syndrome
3. Henoch–Schönlein purpura
4. Microscopic polyangiitis
5. Polyarteritis nodosa
6. Cutaneous vasculitis
7. Temporal arteritis
8. Wegener's granulomatosis
9. Degos
10. Lupus vasculitis.

Other conditions are considered to be the following:

- giant cell arteritis
- polymyalgia rheumatica
- takayasu's arteritis.

Wegener's granulomatosis and some other isolated vasculitis localized in single organs or and polyangiitis may overlap as syndromes.

Diagnosis

Most treatments for vasculitis are dangerous or toxic. Therefore, diagnosis should be clearly established as soon as possible (when possible), with specific target-tissue biopsy. Clinical data and observations may be used to confirm the diagnosis and define the localization of the affected vessels.

Small arteries

Arteriography can be used to evaluate the affected vessels and the localization of the involved segments but angiography — generally used late in the evolution of the condition — only reveals the lumen and often does not give clear information of the structure of the vessel walls.

In temporal arteritis, signs and symptoms may indicate the localization of the lesions. Biopsies should be performed only on selected, well-defined segments (that may be detected, e.g., by high-resolution ultrasound).

As vasculitis can be segmental and lesions (both involving vessels and tissues) often focalized, even a biopsy in a nontarget segment may be inconclusive. Therefore, multiple sampling may be needed. Intimal thickening and arterial wall hypertrophy are seen by high-resolution ultrasound in most arteries and these should be the targets for biopsies.

Laboratory tests are often inconclusive; serum tests for antineutrophil cytoplasmic antibodies (ANCAs) are useful particularly in Wegener's granulomatosis and microscopic polyangiitis. The diagnosis of secondary vasculitis is also complex but clinical history helps.

When the primary cause is known, a biopsy is not always indispensable (e.g., a previous treatment with mesalazine for ulcerative colitis may be found to be a possible initial cause for eosinophilic pneumonia in subjects with suspected Churg–Strauss syndrome). A drug or antigen may be the initial cause in many patients and should be identified. In some cases, vasculitis is secondary to other evident diseases or disorders. The unifying character of vasculitis is the inflammatory process and therefore the possible positive action that corticosteroid may have, sometimes only temporarily.

Ex juvantibus diagnosis (EJD) may confirm the inflammatory cause of the vasculitis before tests may be available. EJD does not necessarily indicate a deficit in a diagnostic process. For example, a patient presenting with retrosternal pain not responding to nitrates but relieved with antacids may benefit by this diagnostic process before definitive tests may be available. The definition *ex juvantibus* in many forms of vasculitis may indicate the general nature of the clinical problem before the availability of tests that may require time to be available or conclusive.

Behçet's syndrome (BE-SY)

Behçet disease (Behçet's syndrome, *Morbus Behçet*, Silk Road disease) may lead to ulceration and other lesions. It has been called Silk Road disease because it is most common and more severe in people originating from countries along the Silk Road, the vast network of ancient trade routes connecting China with the Mediterranean Basin.

The disease appears to be common in Japan, Turkey and Israel, but relatively rare in the USA. It is mainly known in medical terms as Behçet's syndrome. Hulusi Behçet, a Turkish dermatologist, described a disease of inflamed blood vessels in 1937.

BE-SY is considered a relapsing inflammatory multisystem vasculitis. Oral and genital ulcers, ocular inflammation and skin lesions are common features. Blindness, neurological and GI involvement, venous thrombosis and arterial aneurysms are the most clinically important problems.

Diagnosis is mainly clinical, using defined international criteria. The real cause is still unknown but immunological and bacterial or viral origins have been suggested and observed. Hla-b51 is associated with cases from the Mediterranean area, Turkey, Iran, Korea, Japan and China. Behçet's is considered uncommon in the USA.

Vasculitic alterations and thrombosis can be observed at histology. The disease starts usually around 20 years of age and may be equally distributed between sexes (however some sources report a male prevalence). Children with Behçet's have also been observed. Eventually the clinical observations make the diagnosis. Treatment is mainly symptomatic, including corticosteroids for acute or severe manifestations (ocular and neurological manifestations). Immunosuppressants — when there is a strong immunological component — may be used for severe chronic manifestations.

First manifestations may be recurrent, painful oral ulcerations (aphtha-type) stomatitis. Comparable ulcers at the penis, scrotum and vulva may be present and are very painful. Vaginal ulcers tend to cause less pain and are often limited. Ocular disease generally occurs after years: relapsing iridocyclitis is associated to pain, photophobia, hazy vision. Hypopyon with a layer of pus visible in the anterior chamber is specific but not common. Posterior segments may be involved (choroiditis, retinal vasculitis, papillitis decreasing visual acuity). Untreated posterior uveitis may lead to blindness.

Skin lesions

Vesicles, folliculitis, papules, pustules are seen in some 80% of patients. *Erytema nodosum*-like lesions are suggestive of BE-SY; in some 40% of patients, pustular inflammatory reactions to minor trauma (needles), mild, self-limiting arthralgias, neutrophil-mediated arthritis (knees and large joints) in 50% of patients may be observed.

Recurrent superficial or deep venous thrombosis (DVT) may be observed in some 25% of patients and may lead to vena cava obstruction. Involvement of the central nervous system may occur as chronic meningoencephalitis, small-vessel disease with a multiple-sclerosis pattern, and paralyzing, life-threatening brain stem and spinal cord lesions.

Gastrointestinal manifestations are variable from minor abdominal discomfort to real pain and diarrhea with ulcers that may be comparable to the lesions seen in Crohn's disease. A clinical picture of generalized vasculitis may even cause aneurysms or thrombosis in different localizations including the lungs. Focal glomerulonephritis is considered rare and may be asymptomatic.

Diagnosis

BE-SY should be suspected in adults with the following:

- recurrent, oral aphthous ulcers
- unexplained ocular findings
- genital ulcers.

The diagnosis is clinical and may require long periods of observation. International criteria indicate the following for diagnosis:

- recurrent oral ulcers
- two of the following:
  o recurrent genital ulcers
  o eye lesions
  o skin lesions
  o positive pathergy test in absence of any other clinical explanation.

The pathergy test is a papular or pustular reaction to skin puncture with a 20-gauge needle.

Differential diagnosis includes the following:

- reactive arthritis
- Stevens–Johnson syndrome
- systemic lupus erythematosus (SLE)
- Crohn's disease
- ulcerative colitis
- ankylosing spondylitis
- Herpes simplex infections (especially with recurrent aseptic meningitis).

BE-SY has no specific findings excluding other clinical possibilities; it is characterized by its relapsing course and multiple organ involvement. Laboratory tests are nonspecific or characteristic of inflammatory diseases (elevated ESR and $\alpha2$ and γ-globulins, mild leukocytosis).

Prognosis and treatment

BE-SY is chronic but controllable in most cases. Signs and symptoms tend to decrease in intensity over time. Remissions and relapses may last from a week to years even decades. Blindness, caval obstruction, paralysis may complicate more severe cases. Death is possible for neurologic, vascular (aneurysms-thrombosis) or gastrointestinal (GI) involvement.

The treatment is mainly symptomatic. Needle puncture causes more inflammation and skin lesions and should be avoided. Twice daily oral doses of Cochicine 0.5 mg/d decrease the frequency and severity of oral/ genital ulcers. Topical corticosteroid may relieve ocular and oral symptoms. However topical corticosteroids do not change the frequency of relapses.

Patients with severe uveitis or CNS involvement respond to high-dose systemic corticosteroids (prednisone 60–80 mg po bid/d). Posterior uveitis not responding to prednisone can be treated with azathioprine (50–150 mg po once daily or cyclosporine 5 mg/kg po once daily, increased incrementally if needed to 10 mg/kg until a response is observed. Cyclosporine levels should be maintained between 50 and 200 ng/mL. In refractory disease, cyclophosphamide and chlorambucil have been used.

Other treatments according to individual cases include the following:

- interferon alpha
- thalidomide
- pentoxifylline
- etanercept
- infliximab
- PGE1 in case of ischemic lesions and sustained vasospasm.

Churg–Strauss syndrome/disease

In 1951, in New York at Mount Sinai, Drs. J. Churg and L. Strauss defined the Churg–Strauss syndrome (CSS or "allergic granulomatosis"). The syndrome is a medium–small-vessel autoimmune vasculitis, leading to necrosis. CSS is generally characterized by a systemic necrotizing vasculitis in association with granulomas. The average age at onset is around 45 years. CSS is considered rare (possibly three cases per million per year). CSS involves mainly lung blood vessels (it may begin as an apparent, severe type of asthma, resistant to treatments); the gastrointestinal system and peripheral nerves may be involved but the syndrome may also affect the heart, skin and kidneys.

CSS is rare and considered noninheritable and nontransmissible. It was once considered a variant of polyarteritis nodosa (PAN) due to the very similar morphology of the clinical aspects in many cases. CSS has been precipitated by lowering the dose of corticosteroids in patients using leukotriene receptor antagonists for asthma.

Signs/symptoms

Signs/symptoms are apparently similar to PAN (see below). However, the pulmonary involvement is specific, often predominant. The final diagnosis can only be made by biopsy. Nowadays CSS is considered different from PAN, which rarely affects lung vessels.

The diffuse vasculitis involves small and large vessels and it is associated with asthma and eosinophilia. The association with asthma and eosinophilia suggests a form of hypersensitivity. Granulomas tend to grow in vessels and surrounding tissues and the level of blood eosinophilia tends to increase.

Lungs, skin, the cardiovascular system — also including coronary arteries — may be involved. Hypertension may be present; kidneys, the GI system and the peripheral nervous system may be involved and show vasculitis at different levels. Dyspnea, wheezing and cough are common. Chest X-ray shows significant pulmonary involvements and infiltrates. CSS is suspected and defined in patients with symptoms or signs of vasculitis in other organs. Altered complete blood count (CBC) and ANCAs should be evaluated. Some 80% of CSS patients have eosinophils >1,000 cells/μL. Some patients have a positive p-ANCA (ANCA associated to myeloperoxidase). ANCA may differentiate CSS from WEG-Granulomatosis (c-ANCA, reactive mainly to proteinase-3, is usually negative in CSS). Prognosis and treatment are comparable to those for PAN. However, CSS tends to be more responsive to corticosteroids.

Henoch–Schönlein Purpura

Summary

Henoch–Schönlein purpura (HSP or allergic-anaphylactoid purpura) is a type of vasculitis, mostly observed in children and affecting mainly small vessels. This disease is, generally, self-limiting.

Palpable purpura, glomerulonephritis, arthralgias and GI symptoms are usually observed. Corticosteroids tend to improve arthralgia and GI symptoms but without altering the course of HSP. Progressive glomerulonephritis (with blood in urines) may require high-dose corticosteroid or cyclophosphamide. HSP is basically caused by the deposition of IgA-containing immune complexes into the wall of small arteries (skin and other organs) with activation of complement. Possible starters of these processes may include some drugs, food, insect bites and some viruses in upper respiratory tract infection (URI). The typical renal lesions are focal, with segmental areas of proliferative glomerulonephritis.

Signs/symptoms

A sudden, palpable purpura-type rush may be the first sign. The rash involves the extensor surfaces of the feet, arms and a strip across the buttocks (Fig. 1). Initially the lesions may resemble urticaria and soon become indurated and palpable. Different localizations may appear in the following days and weeks.

Fever and polyarthalgia, periarticular tenderness, swelling of wrists, elbows, ankles, knees and hips can be observed in a variable set of symptoms. Abdominal pain or tenderness with colic and melena may be observed. Intussusception may develop in some patients and the stools may be

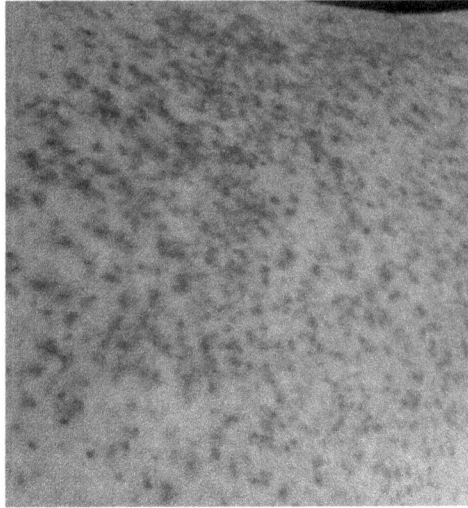

Figure 1. HS purpura, external surface of leg. Girl, age 20. Possible trigger: use of NSAIDs a few weeks before. Blood in urine. Systemic symptoms. Resolution after 6 weeks with corticosteroids. No consequences after 5 years.

positive for occult blood. Blood in the urine may indicate a significant renal involvement.

After about 4–6 weeks, usually, signs/symptoms tend to decrease in intensity but they may recur at least once in most patients after a period of several weeks free of symptoms or problems. In most patients, particularly with the present management and care, the disorder may disappear without consequences. In some patients — particularly if untreated — chronic renal failure may develop in time and therefore some sort of monitoring may be required.

Diagnosis, prognosis and treatment

HSP is suspected, particularly in children, on the basis of typical skin observations. Biopsy of the skin lesions (indicating leukocytoclastic vasculitis with IgA in the vessel walls) is generally diagnostic. Hematuria, proteinuria and RBC casts indicate kidney damage. In patients with significant kidney involvement, a renal biopsy is usually mandatory and may eventually define the diagnosis. Diffuse glomerular involvement may indicate rapidly progressive renal failure.

Treatment is generally symptomatic with the exception of those cases induced by drugs (if the event can be shown). Corticosteroid management (prednisone 2mg/kg) helps to control edema, joint pain and abdominal involvement and generally controls pain in most cases. The long-term effects on the kidney damage is unclear. Immunosuppressive therapy (IV methylprednisolone followed by oral prednisone and cyclophosphamide) may control inflammation in cases with the most severe renal involvement.

Microscopic polyangiitis

Microscopic polyangiitis (MPA) is considered a *pauci-immune systemic necrotizing vasculitis* involving small vessels. It may affect lungs and kidneys. The final diagnosis is only made by biopsy and by measuring ANCAs. The management/treatment is similar to PAN (see below). MPA affects arteries but it may also involve arterioles and venules. Immunocomplexes are not generally involved. This disease is considered more common than PAN but it is still uncommon (possibly 2.4 cases per million). Unlike PAN, MPA may affect pulmonary capillaries and frequently cause glomerulonephritis.

Signs/symptoms

Considered comparable to PAN, MPA may be characterized by cough with dyspnea being more frequent. MPA should be suspected in any patient with evidence of systemic necrotising vasculitis with pulmonary and renal involvement.

Diagnosis

The presence of MPA is only diagnosed with biopsy. It is differentiated from PAN by the absence of immune complex deposition and additional involvement of small vessels (pulmonary capillaries, glomerulonephritis) on biopsy. Lab tests for ANCAs help differentiate MPA from PAN and from Wegener's granulomatosis which can also cause pulmonary and renal vasculitis. ANCAs (those based on the reaction to myeloperoxidase and those that have staining concentrated around and in neutrophilic nuclei: p-ANCA) are most common in PAN.

Prognosis and treatment

Management is similar to the management for PAN. In critically ill patients, e.g., with significant pulmonary hemorrhages, high-dose IV or oral corticosteroids and IV cyclophosphamide (500–750 mg/m^2 once a month for 6 months) have been used. Cases of microscopic polyangiitis in pregnant women have been described.

The management of these cases is particularly complex. Severe cases of MPA presenting with liver dysfunction or preceding rapidly progressive necrotizing glomerulonephritis may require complex monitoring and aggressive management in specialized centers.

Polyarteritis nodosa (polyarteritis, periarteritis nodosa and PAN)

PAN is a systemic necrotizing vasculitis characterized by segmental inflammation and necrosis of medium-sized muscular arteries. Arterial necrosis, thrombosis and occlusion may cause selective tissue ischemia. PAN is considered rare. It occurs most commonly between ages 40 and 50 but can appear at any age. It is considered to be more common in men.

Symptoms and signs are not very specific (fever, weight loss, abdominal pain, neuritis, hypertension and edema). PAN may have an acute or chronic evolution. Unusual combinations of symptoms can be a clue for PAN. A defined diagnosis requires biopsy and/or arteriography. Treatment with corticosteroids and immunosuppressive is often effective.

The initial cause of PAN is generally unknown. Immune mechanisms are often involved. Multiple pathogenic mechanisms may be indicated by the variety of clinical and pathogenic mechanism: 20% of patients have hepatitis B infection. Drugs may be an initial detonating cause. No predisposing antigen has been identified.

Systemic vasculitis similar to PAN is observed in patients with some lymphomas and leukemias. The observed typical lesions are segmental, with necrotising inflammation, medial-adventitial generally occurring at the level of medium-sized arteries. The arterial localizations of PAN are most common at the bifurcations.

These lesions can be present in all stages. Early lesions include PMNs and occasionally eosinophils. Later lesions may include lymphocytes and plasma cells. Intimal proliferation and secondary thrombosis with occlusion generally lead to organ lesions and tissue infarctions with ischemia. Progressive weakening of the muscular components of the vessels walls may cause small localized aneurysms and arterial dissection.

During the healing process, scarring may cause nodular fibrosis of the adventitia and vessel irregularities. Cutaneous, peripheral nerve, hepatic, cardiac and GI involvement are frequently observed. Generally, the pulmonary arteries are not involved. Renal lesions are primarily characterized by glomerular ischemia and infarctions rather than glomerulonephritis. Occasionally, massive hepatic infarction may develop. When these lesions occur, PAN is the determining cause in some 50% of cases. Focal areas of hepatic capsular vasculitis are more common.

Signs/symptoms

PAN may mimic several clinical conditions. In each patient, there may be a predominant localization in one organ or system. Acute or chronic evolutions are possible: a subacute clinical evolution may become rapidly progressive and even fatal after months. PAN may also be a chronic, slow and debilitating disease.

The location and severity of the arterial lesions and the consequent, secondary circulatory impairment define signs and symptoms. The most common initial complaints are fever (85% of patients), abdominal pain (65%), peripheral neuropathy (often mononeuritis multiplex) (50%), weakness and/or weight loss are seen in 45% of patients.

Hypertension is seen in many patients (60%), and symptoms such as edema, oliguria and uremia are also present in patients with renal involvement. Right-upper quadrant abdominal tenderness is considered common. Diffuse or localized abdominal pain, nausea, vomiting, bloody diarrhea may be an expression of organ ischemia, bowel or gallbladder perforation, intussusception and even peritonitis.

GI hemorrhage or retroperitoneal bleeding may also occur and should be always considered as a possibility in these patients. Angina may be seen in some 25% of patients but asymptomatic coronary disease is more common. CNS involvement may cause headaches and even seizures in a small number of patients.

Muscular problems (e.g., myalgias) may be associated to areas of focal ischemic myositis and arthralgias are considered common. Well-defined arthritis of large joints may occur. Skin lesions, including palpable purpura, palpable subcutaneous nodules along the course of affected arteries and irregular areas of necrosis may occur in some patients. Orchitis and testicular pain are also possible.

When small and medium arteries are involved hypertension, oliguria and uremia and other *renal symptoms* may be present. Urinary alterations with hematuria and no cellular casts can be seen. The course of hypertension may be faster. Renal artery and kidney circulation aneurysms may rupture and cause hematomas or renal infarcts with lumbar pain and hematuria. Renal ischemia and infarctions may produce renal failure.

Diagnosis

PAN is suspected in patients with unexplained fever, abdominal pain, indications of renal failure or sudden hypertension. Unexplained arthralgias, muscle tenderness, subcutaneous nodules, purpuric skin rashes, pain in the abdomen or extremities are also considered indications of PAN. Rapidly developing hypertension is a particularly important observation.

The definitive diagnosis is usually indicated by a combination of clinical and laboratory features, particularly if the illness is multisystemic. A systemic illness associated with peripheral, usually multiple, neuritis involving major nerve trunks (e.g., radial, peroneal sciatic) with asymmetric or symmetric distribution (mononeuritis multiplex) also suggests PAN.

Necrotising arteritis seen on biopsy or typical aneurysms in medium-sized arteries can be also seen on angiograms or revealed by ultrasound.

Blind biopsy is considered useless. PAN has a diffuse distribution with a focal expression and can be diagnosed by selective, aimed biopsy. Skin, subcutaneous tissue, sural nerve and muscle may be preferred to kidney or liver biopsy for an initial diagnosis. Electromyography and nerve conduction studies help select the location of the biopsy.

A testicular biopsy (when microscopic lesions at this site are present) is rarely diagnostic. Renal biopsy (in patients with renal disease) and liver biopsy (in patients with abnormal liver function tests) are usually appropriate if other involved sites fail to produce a bioptic diagnosis. Even without a firm tissue diagnosis, abdominal angiography is considered diagnostic when typical aneurysms are seen in renal, hepatic and celiac vessels.

All laboratory tests are considered not very specific or not diagnostic. Leukocytosis in the range of 20,000–40,000/μL is shown in 80% of patients. Proteinuria can be present in 60% of patients, microscopic hematuria in 40%. These are the most frequent abnormalities detected by laboratory tests.

Thrombocytosis, marked elevation of ESR and anemia caused by blood loss or renal failure can be also seen. Hypoalbuminemia, elevated serum immunoglobulins can occur in a significant number of patients. Measurement of autoantibodies may differ from other connective tissue disease. Antibodies are rarely present in PAN. In most patients, liver enzymes can be, at least, mildly elevated.

Prognosis

Untreated disease is usually fatal, often ending in kidney or liver failure, failure of other organs (including GI) or aneurysms rupture. Without treatment, some 70% of patients with PAN may theoretically die in 12 months and 90% within 5 years. With present management, however, these numbers are now being challenged. Oliguria and hypertension indicate advanced disease. Renal failure causes death in over 65% of patients. Potentially fatal hospital or opportunistic infections may occur.

A long-term remission may be achieved with aggressive treatment, but management and therapy must be tailored to clinical evidence and strongly individualized. Possible offending agents (including drugs), if suspected or known, should be eliminated. The risk of infection is generally increased; the associated infections should be aggressively treated.

Treatment

High-dose corticosteroids (e.g., prednisone 60 mg po once daily) may prevent progression and induce partial or near-complete remission in about 30% of patients. The response may vary in different patients. When long-term treatment is needed, adverse effects, including hypertension (which may aggravate or accelerate kidney damage), must be carefully managed. The daily dose of corticosteroids should be progressively reduced if and when improvement is achieved (considering a decrease in fever and particularly in ESR).

Improvements in cardiac and renal function, improvement in neuropathy, disappearance of cutaneous lesions, decreased pain) also indicate the need to reduce the load of treatment. Long-term hyperadrenocorticism can be minimized by giving corticosteroids in single morning doses every other day. This type of administration can be effective as a maintenance therapy but is rarely successful as an early treatment.

Immunosuppressants are used if patients do not respond to corticosteroids during the first few weeks of therapy or if the doses of corticosteroids needed to control symptoms become too high (however this applies to most patients). Cyclophosphamide 2–3 mg/kg po once a day may be administered. The dose should be adjusted to keep the WBC count at >300/μL. Hydration is needed to decrease the risks of bladder hemorrhage, cystitis or bladder cancer. Pulse IV cyclophosphamide may be less toxic but may also be less effective.

Management

Signs/symptoms and complications (e.g., hypertension), fluid management, treatment of renal insufficiency and anemia require a complex multitreatment plan. Surgical intervention for GI involvement (including intussusception or mesenteric artery thrombosis, bowel and/or visceral infarction) are measures to control an emergency but do not treat the problems. In patients with hepatitis B- or C-associated vasculitis, interferon alpha and other newer antiviral drugs (e.g., lamivudine) may be effective.

Hepatitis B-related PAN

Treatment should control and suppress inflammation rapidly; the following task is to eliminate the virus and induce seroconversion via plasma exchange. Corticosteroids are used for a few weeks. Lamivudine 100 mg/d po once a day is used for not more than 6 months. In case of renal insufficiency, the dose is lower.

Plasma exchanges are used three times a week in the first 3 weeks and then twice a week for a further 2 weeks followed by once a week until hepatitis B e-antigen (HBeAg) converts to hepatitis B e-antibody (anti-HBe) or until clinical recovery is stable for 2–3 months.

This management plan may not improve survival in comparison with immunosuppressive therapy. It may only be that the risk of complications from hepatitis B may be reduced, avoiding side effects of long-term administration of corticosteroids and immunosuppressants.

Conventional treatment with corticosteroids and cytotoxic immuno-suppressants (e.g., cyclophosphamide) is effective in the short term but it does not prevent recurrent episodes, chronic hepatitis and cirrhosis as the hepatitis virus could still be present.

Predominantly cutaneous vasculitis (PCV)

The condition known as primarily cutaneous vasculitis (PCV, leukocyto-clastic vasculitis, hypersensitivity vasculitis) affects mainly small cutane-ous vessels, causing skin lesions. Common causes of PCV may include serum sickness, infections such as hepatitis C, some cancers, rheumato-logic or other autoimmune conditions/disorders. Hypersensitivity to drugs is also considered a cause in some cases. Systemic vasculitis is possible but generally is less severe than with the systemic necrotising forms of vasculitis.

Immune complex deposition probably mediates vessel inflammation. Neutrophil fragments and debris (leukocytoclasis) within/around small vessels may cause leukocytoclastic vasculitis. PCV may cause a variety of skin lesions (most commonly a palpable purpura), and there are often systemic symptoms (such as polyarthralgia, fever).

The diagnosis should be made by skin biopsy. Treatments are determined by the identification of the underlying cause. If no apparent cause can be identified and severe, systemic vasculitis develops, patients should receive corticosteroids and sometimes, immunosuppressants. The management is very individualized and tends to follows symptoms and organs, localizations: it is broadly comparable or similar to the management used for PAN.

Temporal arteritis

Temporal arteritis (giant cell arteritis, cranial arteritis) is a chronic inflammatory disease of large blood vessels (carotid artery branches, occurring mainly in older adults). Association with polymyalgia rheumatica is considered common. Frequent signs/symptoms include headaches, visual disturbances, temporal artery tenderness, pain in the jaw muscles while chewing. Fever, weight loss and malaise or fatigue are also common; ERS is usually very high.

The diagnosis is generally made by a selective biopsy (on arterial sites selected by ultrasound and showing thickening and infiltration) when possible. Management: The treatment includes high-dose corticosteroids; it is usually very effective and may prevent visual loss. The specific etiology and pathogenesis of this condition are still unknown. It is considered rare in patients younger than 55 and appears to be more common in women. The prevalence appears to be higher in North-Europeans (15–25 cases/100,000).

Pathology

Vasculitis may be localized, multifocal or widespread, most often involving temporal, cranial or other carotid artery branches (prevalently in the territory of the external carotid) and even the coronary arteries. Arteries with a prevalence of elastic tissue components are affected more often.

The granulomatous inflammation primarily involves the media. Lymphocytes, epithelioid cells, and often giant cells may be observed.

Elastic components are progressively disrupted, the intima is markedly thickened (this is visible by ultrasound) with lumen narrowing and eventually obstruction that may produce distal ischemia.

Signs/symptoms

Symptoms are normally related to the distribution of the arteritis. Typically, severe, sometimes throbbing headache (with temporal–occipital localization), associated to visual disturbances (amaurosis fugax, diplopia, scotomata, ptosis and blurred vision) and pain at the masseter and temporalis muscles on chewing (jaw claudication) is observed. Most patients report pain on the scalp or when combing. Systemic symptoms may include fever, malaise, weight loss and sweating; some patients may also present with symptoms corresponding to polymyalgia rheumatica (PMR), carpal tunnel syndrome, radiculopathy and rarely, pulse deficits comparable to Takayasu's arteritis.

Blindness (ischemic optic neuropathy) may occur in <10% of patients but it can be sudden and irreversible. Some swelling, tenderness with a diffuse nodularity over the temporal arteries or bruits over large vessels may also be present but again, uncertainty may remain as to whether it is only temporal arteritis.

Diagnosis

The diagnosis is clinical and confirmed by a biopsy of the temporal artery if clinically needed. Temporal arteritis may be suspected in patients <55, with signs/symptoms compatible with ischemia related to neck–head arteries, with pain on chewing, newly onset headaches and tender temporal arteries.

Associated symptoms of PMR may increase the possibility of temporal arteritis. A possible elevation in ESR and C-reactive protein should be evaluated. ESR can be markedly elevated (>100 mm/h; Westergren) during the most active phases. It can be normal in some patients as C-reactive protein. Normochromic–normocytic anemia is often present. Leukocytosis is frequent but nonspecific. Serum alkaline phosphatase may be elevated and polyclonal hyperglobulinemia may be observed.

As indicated, clinical diagnosis should be confirmed by a direct, selective biopsy. Vasculitis may also involve small branches of the temporal arteries. Bilateral biopsy, removal of damages arterial segments (>2 cm) may be indicated and may relieve some symptoms. Temporal arteritis may require a diagnostic biopsy even after corticosteroid treatment. However, a biopsy and the treatments should not be delayed. In subjects with pulse deficits, an evaluation by ultrasound may be needed while arteriography is rarely necessary.

Treatment

The treatment can start as soon as temporal arteritis is suspected even if the biopsy is delayed. The treatment prevents serious complications as blindness. Prednisone 60 mg po once daily is used for 2–4 weeks. If symptoms improve, prednisone can be tampered gradually according to individual responses, usually by 2–5 mg/d per week until reaching 10–20 mg/po once a day; the therapy may be followed by 1 mg/d per week thereafter.

ESR tends to decrease with treatment but full normalization is not necessary. Therefore, prednisone should not be increased on the basis of ESR. When signs/symptoms flare with tampering, the dose can be slightly increased again.

Some patients may stop prednisone within 1 year but they may require small doses for years. Azathioprine and methotrexate may be used in some patients but may have unacceptable results or adverse effects. Evidence of efficacy with these products is limited and treatments may be balanced against important side effects. Infusion of PGE1 in some patients may safely improve symptoms and decrease the level of inflammation.

Wegener's granulomatosis

Wegener's granulomatosis (WG) is considered uncommon; the disease usually begins with localized granulomatous inflammation of the upper or lower respiratory tract mucosa. It may progress to generalized necrotizing granulomatous vasculitis and glomerulonephritis. Patients may have recurrent nasal discharge or bleeding, lung nodules, infiltrates and hypertension or glomerulonephritis as manifestations of systemic vasculitis.

The diagnosis is generally made with a biopsy and management is generally based on corticosteroid treatment and cyclophosphamide. The causes of WG are unknown. Immunologic mechanisms may be involved in different phases and with a complex interaction. WG occurs in about 1/25,000 people, most commonly in the Caucasian population. It may occur at any age; the mean age at onset is around 40 years.

Pathophysiology

WG is characterized by a necrotising vasculitis of the small arteries and veins and by the presence of intra or extravascular granulomas. Multinucleated giant cells are generally present, particularly in the lungs. WG affects all organs but the respiratory tract and kidney are most often, specifically affected. Nasopharyngeal inflammation and granulomas may evolve into local necrosis.

The lungs develop infiltrates and can develop multiple cavities. Kidney lesions may begin as focal glomerulitis progressing to diffuse glomerulonephritis. Necrotising renal vasculitis is possible but kidney granulomas are uncommon.

Signs/symptoms

The onset of WG may be acute or subclinical. The full spectrum of WG may take years to become clinically clear. Initial complaints are localized to the upper respiratory tract with purulent or bloody nasal discharge, paranasal sinusitis pain, nasal mucosal ulcerations (with consequent secondary bacterial infections). Serous or purulent otitis media, recurring cough, hemoptysis can all be present. Nasal granulomas may resemble sinusitis and can give the nasal mucosa a red, raised granulomatous appearance and a friable texture. Nasal perforations may occur.

Fever, malaise, anorexia weight loss, migratory polyarthritis, granulomatous or leukocytoclastic vasculitic skin lesions, nasolacrimal duct obstruction, retrobulbar granulomas with proptosis and episcleritis may be observed. Chondritis of the ear pinna and myocardial infarction (MI) from coronary localizations of the vasculitis may occur.

A disseminated vasculitis may occur with pulmonary symptoms (dyspnea, hemophthisis) necrotizing inflammatory skin lesions, renovascular hypertension and kidney failure. Occasionally, the disease remains limited to the lungs. Renal involvement is the hallmark of generalized disease. Important anemia causes fatigue and weakness.

Diagnosis

WG is suspected in patients with the following:

1. chronic unexplained respiratory symptoms,
2. involvement of other systems (kidney).

ANCAs require evaluation. Leukocytosis and anemia are common and may be important. Eosinophilia is considered rare. ESR is elevated in case of active inflammation and mild hypergammaglobulinemia may be present. ANCA with a predominant reaction to proteinase-3 (c-ANCA) is present in 90% of patients with kidney and respiratory involvement (70% of patients without kidney involvement). ANCA is highly specific for WG but c-ANCA is not considered diagnostic. Biopsy should confirm necrotizing granulomatous vasculitis in subjects with respiratory manifestations and glomerulonephritis.

Nasal and sinus tissue are the most accessible but often these samples are not very diagnostic. The most suspicious lesion should be the target of the biopsy. Lung biopsy is the most possible site to obtain a positive biopsy. The biopsy should not be delayed in the case of pulmonary involvement: open thoracotomy provides the best access to the affected tissue.

Kidney involvement may be assessed with urinalysis (proteinuria, hematuria and RBC casts). Renal biopsy may be needed if glomerulonephritis is suspected (hematuria and proteinuria) especially if serum creatinine is increased. Renal biopsy does not show granulomas and therefore is, generally, less diagnostic than other biopsies.

Differential diagnosis should be made with the following:

• *PAN*: PAN rarely affects the lungs and is ruled out by granulomatous findings on biopsy.

- *CSS and MPA*: The difference is made considering the absence of nasal involvement and ANCA reactive mainly to myeloperoxidase (p-ANCA). In this condition, there is significant eosinophilia. RA cannot be diagnosed as 50% of WeGr have high RA.

Blood culture and clinical manifestations may be needed to exclude infective endocarditis. Infective endocarditis, SLE (differentiated by the presence of antinuclear antibodies and in some cases, slow serum complement) can be considered in the differential diagnosis. Slow infection due to fungi should be also considered.

Prognosis and treatment

Limited disease may have nasal and pulmonary lesions with little or no systemic involvement. Pulmonary manifestations may improve or worsen spontaneously. In subjects with the complete syndrome, manifestations usually progress rapidly to renal failure once the diffuse vasculitis begins. Untreated, diffuse vasculitis tends to be rapidly fatal. The prognosis is dramatically improved by treatment with immunosuppressants.

Early diagnosis and treatment are crucial, because a high remission rate is now possible. Renal complication can be avoided or controlled with the appropriate management. Cyclophosphamide (2 mg/kg po, once a day) is considered the drug of choice. Careful hydration is needed to decrease the risks of bladder hemorrhage, cystitis and bladder cancer. Corticosteroids, which reduce vasculitic edema, are given concurrently (e.g., prednisone 1 mg/kg po, once a day).

After 2–3 months, prednisone is tapered until the patient is maintained solely on oral cyclophosphamide (long-term IV dosing of cyclophosphamide appears to be less effective in maintaining remission). Cyclophosphamide is given for more than 1 year after the clinical remission. Daily dose is then decreased by 25 mg between 2 and 3 months.

Disease activity can be assessed by symptoms, signs, chest x-rays, urinalysis and renal function tests. c-ANCA may normalize but is not the most important measure to follow. Patients achieving remission on cyclophosphamide may be maintained on treatment with methotrexate using less than 20–25 po once a week.

Azathioprine is considered a less effective alternative. To prevent secondary pneumonia, long-term prophylactic treatment with trimethoprim-sulfamethoxazole (160 + 800 mg po once a day; Bactrim) could be associated. Complete, long-term remission may be achieved in many patients, even when there is an advanced active disease.

Kidney transplantation may be an important option in renal failure. An increased incidence of solid tumors and bladder cancer after many years may be associated to the chronic use of high-dose cyclophosphamide. Therefore, adequate screening is important for these patients.

Degos disease (malignant atrophic papulosis)

Degos disease is an extremely rare vasculopathy that affects the lining of the medium and small veins and arteries, resulting in occlusion (with block of some arteries) and tissue infarction. Robert Degos recognized this conditions as a clinical entity in 1942.

The blood vessels affected include those forming the skin, the gastrointestinal tract and the central nervous system. Lesions may cause bowel ischemia (mesenteric ischemia or ischemic colitis), chronic skin lesions, ocular lesions, strokes, spinal lesions, mononeuritis multiplex, epilepsy, headaches and cognitive disorders. Pleural or pericardial effusions have also been reported.

The outcome of Degos disease can be fatal with an average survival of 2–3 years. Some patients may have a benign, slow form (Degos acanthoma) which affects only the skin. There are possibly less than 50 living patients at present worldwide. Fewer than 200 have been reported in the medical literature but possibly many cases are not recognized or diagnosed considering the rarity of the condition.

Treatment options are limited, consist mainly of antiplatelet prophylaxis or anticoagulants and are individualized on the basis of the occurring symptoms. Also, immunosuppressants can be used. The effects of treatments are generally limited to case reports. It has been suggested that Degos is not a separate disorder but the final result of several vascular systemic disorders or conditions.

Lupus vasculitis

Lupus vasculitis is one of the numerous polymorphic complications that can arise from the chronic autoimmune inflammatory disease generally defined as lupus. Vasculitis occurs when white blood cells attack small and large blood vessels, causing chronic inflammation. The damage produced by lupus vasculitis ranges from minor skin lesions to severe organ damage caused by the destruction of tissue around those organs. This condition is usually diagnosed clinically and with blood tests, although a biopsy may be used depending on the affected areas.

Management

Treatment of this vasculitis generally begins with cortisone-based medications to which cytotoxic drugs are then added in more severe cases.

Vasculitis generally is related to antigens that cause an allergic reaction within the blood vessel walls. Antibodies bond to the antigen and attract white blood cells to the affected vessel segment. In this form of lupus, white blood cells accumulate in the vessel walls, causing blood vessel wall inflammation. The damage produced by the inflammation can be minor to small blood vessels, or capillaries (these may break, causing red or purple dots on the skin, usually painless). Depending on the severity of the inflammation and its location, the problems caused by lupus vasculitis can become more severe. Inflammation can narrow the vessel lumen, causing reduced perfusion. Arterial and venous blood clots may be observed.

Tissues surrounding the inflamed vessels may necrose leading to gangrene. Serious issues can arise when the vasculitis affects major organs. Vision loss due to retinal damage, pneumonia-like symptoms caused by vasculitis near lung vessels, and brain complications (headaches, seizures, or strokes) are all possible. Commonly associated with this condition are joint problems, with aching, swelling or arthritis.

The diagnosis of lupus vasculitis usually comes from blood tests (white and red blood cells, presence of autoantibodies). Depending on the main location of the vasculitis, CT scans may be diagnostic. Tissue biopsy can also definitively diagnose lupus vasculitis. Treatment of this condition may not be necessary if the problem is limited to the minor bleeding or red or purple spots caused by capillaries breaking. More severe cases often require corticosteroid. Cytotoxic drugs can also be used on the basis of symptoms and localizations.

Takayasu's arteritis: Observations

Takayasu's arteritis (TA) (also known as pulseless disease, occlusive thromboaortopathy, aortic arch syndrome) is an inflammatory disease of unknown origin affecting the aorta and its branches, occurring most often in young women and adolescents. It causes asymmetry of pulses and signs/symptoms associated to arterial obstruction. Diagnosis is made by clinical evaluation, by ultrasound, arteriography or MRI.

The management is based on the localization of the problems; generally, corticosteroids are used when the inflammatory component is important (elevated ESR); severe distal ischemia can be managed very effectively (if there is ischemia) with PGE1 infusions. These infusions may also improve optic ischemia and ischemic symptoms associated to specific organs (kidney) leading to severe complications.

Specific vascular interventions may be needed using angioplasty or stents or open surgery in case of severe, segmental obstructive disease. Embolization may also occur and it may be prevented using anticoagulants as appropriate. TA is considered a rare observation. Reported worldwide epidemiological surveys indicate that TA is more common in Asians. Females are eight times more likely to have this condition. The age of onset of TA may be as low as 15 years and may go up to 30 years.

Progressive inflammation and deposition of several inflammatory and thrombotic products into the arterial wall may narrow, not segmentally, vessel lumen and may eventually cause thrombosis with full obstruction. Late stages of TA include alterations of arterial walls that may lead to aneurysmal dilatation and ruptures.

Signs/symptoms

Half of all patients who develop TA initially develop general signs of inflammation such as malaise, fever, night sweats, weight loss, arthralgia and fatigue. This phase may gradually subside and is followed by a more chronic stage characterized by focal vascular symptoms resulting from ischemia of aortic branches, usually in its arch and at the thoracic regions.

The other some 50% of patients tend to have only focal, localized symptoms. These may include TIA, strokes, syncope, transient visual disturbances (sudden loss of vision) caused by TIAs in the carotid system and in the vertebral arteries.

Pain with the use of an arm (on effort) may be a significant symptom. Muscular atrophy may affect arms and even the face. Bruits may be present over narrowed stenotic arteries. The obstruction of the descending and abdominal aorta may cause claudication or severe vascular disease and renal flow alterations that may be associated to renovascular hypertension (sometimes severe and not easily treatable).

TA may cause also coronary inflammation (eventually determining angina or MI) and infrequently, aortic insufficiency. These sequelae of localized vascular blocks and hypertension (associated to kidney hypoperfusion) may become fatal or, progressively, cause heart failure.

Rarely, pulmonary artery obstruction may lead to pulmonary hypertension. Signs of arterial obstruction may be seen only in advanced stages. Pulses may be very weak or absent with absent or nondetectable brachial arteries to measure blood pressure (BP).

Unless coarctation is present, these pulses, contrast with the generally brick pulses and normal BP in the legs. If the arm vessels are severely affected systemic BP can only be measured in the legs. Nowadays patients are occasionally diagnosed (or screened) by ultrasound years before they become symptomatic (but if the patient actually has TA, it may be difficult to define).

Diagnosis

Ultrasound may show homogeneous, diffuse arterial wall thickening (not atherosclerotic plaques).

Ischemic signs/symptoms

The observation that young Asian women may have TA more often is not very helpful in most clinical contexts. Bruits, asymmetry of pulses and pressure discrepancies are also suggestive of TA but are late signs. The confirmation is generally made by angiography, generally to be performed when an invasive intervention is planned.

Stenosis, obstruction, lumen irregularities, poststenotic dilations, aneurysms tend to have a specific nonatherosclerotic pattern and, generally, are observed in younger subjects. Laboratory tests may be nonspecific and often are not needed unless subjects are in a strong inflammatory storm. If an initial "trigger" condition or disease anemia is present, an increased WBC count and a higher ESR may be considered but are not diagnostic.

Case 1. Lupus vasculitis; "peripheral TIAs" from microembolization. The microembolization was from a possible proximal source (thrombotic, complex plaque at the femoral artery).
Symptoms: Acute, vivid pain, skin necrosis.
Diagnosis: Clinical.
Treatment: PGE1 infusions and LMW heparin. At the moment of the final episode: patient in treatment with corticosteroids in a remission phase. Several episodes of peripheral microembolization had been observed by the patient and diagnosed as "vasculitis". After treatment, antiplatelet agents were added to the treatment. Microembolization did not recur.

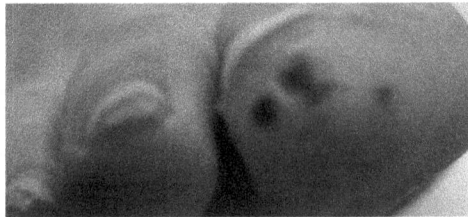

8

Extracranial Carotid Artery
and Cerebrovascular Disease

Introduction

Cerebrovascular symptoms are often caused by embolization from a complex plaque; thrombosis may also occur blocking the inflow to the brain. Possibly, only some 25% of all events are clinically apparent as TIAs or strokes. Repeated, subclinical embolization may cause progressive cerebral damage and atrophy. Around 80% of the emboli may originate from irregular plaques with some thrombotic appositions at the carotid bifurcations. These lesions are often surgically accessible.

Transcranial Doppler studies indicate that embolization can be documented in some 20% of patients with >50% stenosis and irregular plaques. The incidence of embolization appears to be more frequent in symptomatic patients after a stroke or transient deficits. Microembolization of multiple small fragments may progressively occlude distal cerebral arteries.

Acute neurological dysfunctions may include unilateral, contralateral motor or sensory loss, aphasia, dysarthria, amaurosis. When symptoms last less than 24 h, the event is defined as a TIA. If symptoms persist, the event is defined as stroke or cerebrovascular accident or attack (CVA). The distinction is not always simple or completely correct.

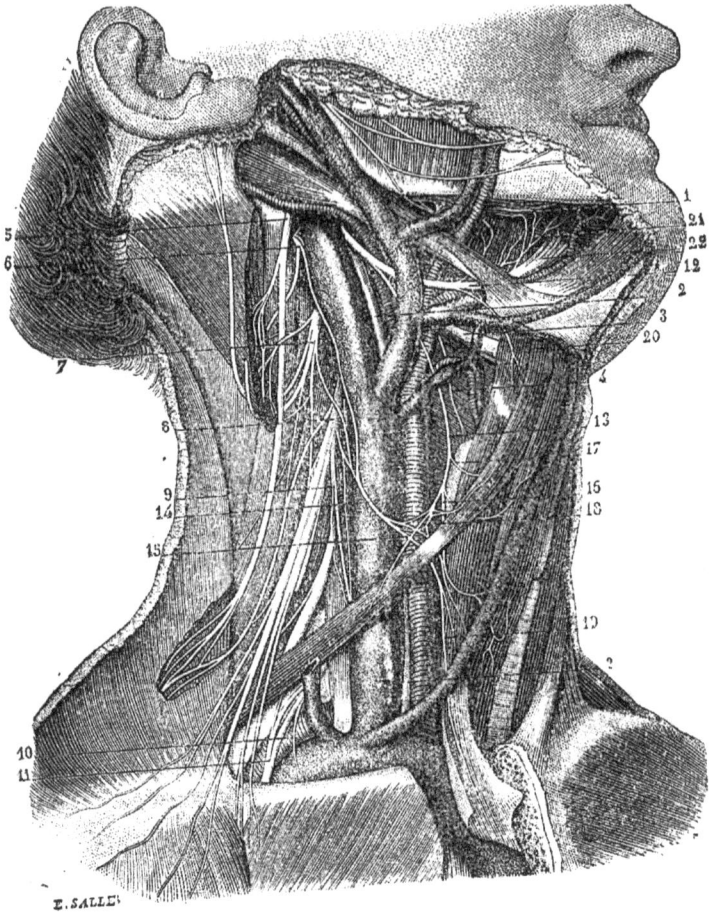

E.SALLE

Embolization into the ophthalmic artery circulation (ipsilateral) may cause amaurosis fugax (temporary blindness) or a more permanent lesion. Emboli may be visible in the retina. Carotid artery lesions are usually localized at the bifurcation, often opposite to the origin of the internal carotid. The bifurcation causes a more turbulent flow predisposing to changes in shear stress and to the development of atherosclerotic lesions.

Without treatment, some 25% of TIA patients develop a stroke with permanent lesions and more that 70% of patients with stenosis may develop a permanent neurological deficit in 2 years. By removing the plaque, or controlling its growth and structure, the risk of events can be reduced to less than 10% per year.

Signs/symptoms

The presence of a bruit is associated with advanced lesions but most patients have no bruit. Stroke and TIAs often occur in the territory of the anterior or middle cerebral artery. Symptoms are generally related to the affected areas, to the size of embolization/infarction and to the presence of collateral flow. Cerebral hypoperfusion (sudden lowering of pressure) may also cause TIAs and visual problems. In symptomatic patients, stroke risk is generally related to the degree of stenosis and to the types of structure of the plaques.

Acute, unstable, neurological deficits may be caused by multiple TIAs — presenting as strokes in evolution — with variable neurological deficits: these conditions are often associated to high degrees of stenosis or to a long, large, complex, unstable plaque. Urgent treatment is needed in these patients. Even with anticoagulation, the deficits may worsen and become permanent in hours.

After a major stroke, either with recovery or residual deficits, patients may suffer from another stroke. After a large infarct, during the recovery and healing period, it is better to prevent hemorrhages into the necrotic (and surrounding edematous) areas.

The vertebro-basilar circulation is less frequently affected by embolization. Situations of hypoperfusion are the most frequent pathology. Flow reduction, drop attacks, sensory symptoms, often bilateral (vertigo, diplopia, dizziness) may be present. Symptoms may be less evident than those caused by plaques in the carotid circulation. Bruits are less frequent in this vascular sector. A careful neurological evaluation is essential.

Diagnosis

Ultrasound

Color duplex show flow alterations and high-resolution scans define plaque conformation, surface and composition; their structure can be defined in minutes. Plaque morphology and stability appear to be as important as stenosis. Homogeneous plaques with a significant (>50% of the area) fibrotic-collagen component (whiter on ultrasound) are more stable than darker plaques without a fibrotic component. The definition of the density and homogeneity of the plaque gives a significant clinical value to ultrasound.

An evaluation of "plaque factors" indicates that the increase in size and length, and in echolucency of the plaque, a decrease in homogenicity and density (softer or blacker plaques on ultrasound) make the plaque more dangerous and prone to embolize. The "black", echolucent component has almost the same density of blood and may be thrombus which may embolize or occlude the artery. The white, fibrotic component (mostly collagen) tends to be more stable and less prone to cause events.

Intracranial/transcranial ultrasound and duplex scanning also offer a view and measurements of intracranial flow and a visual of the main arteries in the brain. The test is usually combined with carotid-vertebral scanning to have a complete evaluation of the system and a possible estimate of the tolerance the brain may have to an occlusion (during possible surgery).

CT and CT angiography

Simple CT — without contrast — is used as the first approach after a TIA or a stroke to exclude the presence of masses, hematomas and to detect significant infarcts. CT angio is a second level investigation; it evaluates the degree of stenosis at the carotid bifurcations and visualizes the aortic arch. Additional elements can also be assessed (proximal, supraaortic vessels and intracerebral vessels).

MR and MRA

MR and MRA (angio) also show the morphology of the ischemic areas and the surrounding areas affected by edema. The software for cerebral MR often shows info that are not always relevant to the acute cerebrovascular problems and the excess in info may be distracting.

Cerebral arteriography

Cerebral arteriography is now performed less frequently in symptomatic and asymptomatic patients. It shows details when noninvasive investigations are not satisfactory (e.g., in calcified arteries) and indicates the possibilities of angioplasty/stenting.

Cerebral arteriography is invasive and may expose some patients to a significant risk of stroke (0.5–1%) or to contrast side effects.

Management

Stroke risk is high after TIAs; the global risk is reduced to previous levels if patients are asymptomatic for 6 months after the episode. Early intervention (thrombolysis, endarterectomy or stenting) may be indicated or mandatory if surgery is possible, available and at low risk. Antiplatelet agents are considered important to prevent new events. Some agents (clopidogrel) are not generally used just before surgery. The aggressive control of cardiovascular risk factors is important. After a complete stroke, the timing for surgery is important if intervention is possible.

Carotid endarterectomy

Endarterectomy reduces strokes from 26% to 9% at 2 years (according to NASCET). However, in this and other comparable carotid studies, the study patients were in specific — highly qualified — institutions; all had a high degree of stenosis; all these studies have been done a few years ago.

With a stenosis <50%, benefits may be limited and treatment should be individualized. Asymptomatic stenosis studies (asymptomatic carotid atherosclerosis study (ACAS) and asymptomatic carotid surgery trial (ACST)) show that stroke incidence is reduced from 12% to 6% with carotid endarterectomy vs the best medical management in a follow up of 6 years.

This study also included institutions with high standards and results are not always replicable. ACAS also indicated there were no benefits or limited results in women (possibly the carotid is too small and the disease, when detected, is more advanced).

Results with medical management are now more advanced; the disease is generally discovered on average 10 years earlier than it previously was; therefore, if we were compare medical and surgical management results now, it could be different from these earlier pivotal studies. After complete occlusion, generally no surgery is advised.

Angioplasty/stenting

Angioplasty or stenting of the carotid bifurcation may produce comparable results with a lower complication rate in comparison with endarterectomy. Protection with specific devices (against embolization) during surgery reduces complication rates during these procedures. Treatment with clopidogrel after stenting (e.g., for 6 weeks) appears to limit new episodes of embolization. Apparently, there are more strokes with stenting than after endarterectomy, whereas myocardial infarctions have been observed more often after endarterectomy.

Both women and men over the age of 70 appear to have worse results with stenting. Younger subjects have much better results. Also, stenting is better for almost-occlusive lesions localized at the origin of the arch vessels and in subjects with recurrent stenosis after treatment. Stenting can be more effective than endarterectomy when anatomy is more complicated, after radiotherapy or in subjects with higher distal lesions, not surgically accessible and when a carotid lesion needs to be treated before coronary surgery.

Results of treatment

The rate of complications for endarterectomy (after strokes) should be below 2–7%. Higher rates may be expected in case of contralateral stenosis or in redo cases, in almost-occlusion (>95% stenosis), when surgery is possible, or in more complex cases. Asymptomatic stenosis tends to produce low rates of complications with surgery.

The death rate for all cases should be below 1%. The risk of strokes should be always compared to the risk of surgery. Temporary nerve injury is possible in <10% of patients causing speech problems, face–mouth asymmetry, earlobe numbness or dysphagia. Less than 2% of these deficits are permanent.

In recurrent cases of stenosis, complications tend to be more frequent and results are often better with stenting. The use of a carotid patch, increasing the amplitude of the lumen, reduces the incidence of restenosis. Restenosis (with a regular but narrowed lumen) could be 5–10% after 5 years; it is possibly less frequent with stenting.

9

Subclavian Steal, Takayasu, Internal Carotid Dissection and Fibromuscular Dysplasia

Subclavian steal

Reversal flow through the vertebral arteries due to more proximal occlusion or stenosis of the subclavian artery may steal blood from the brain, causing symptoms. The syndrome appears to be less common now. Angiography shows the anatomical picture; events are rare and temporary.

Symptomatology

Fatigue is felt at the affected arm and this is a symptom considered more common than those of a neurological nature. The treatment for SST is generally a bypass graft from the common carotid to the subclavian artery, distally to the main lesion or a direct transposition of the subclavian artery beyond the level of the lesion, to the side of the common carotid artery.

Takayasu (giant cell arteritis)

Originally, this uncommon condition was described as an obliterative arteriopathy affecting the aortic arch vessels, mainly in younger women and often causing blindness. The pararenal aorta and the pulmonary arteries may be also involved. There is diffuse, linear thickening affecting the arteries, particularly carotids, not localized at the bifurcations.

Corticosteroids, anticoagulants, cyclophosphamide and a severe risk reduction management may arrest, and in some patients reverse, the disease that is now, generally, diagnosed years before a full occlusion of the arteries as seen in the original descriptions.

Operative treatment options are more limited than in pure, typical atherosclerosis with very localized lesions and are not considered during the inflammatory phase. Invasive methods are possible and could be more effective, when the disease is quiescent or in remission, on a very individual basis.

Internal carotid dissection

Internal carotid dissection is rare; it may occur in adults during exercise or as a consequence of a neck trauma. The lesion is associated to intimal tear, generally, at the distal end of the carotid bulb. These lesions are generally acute and may be associated to a trauma in different conditions (including indirect trauma) or may develop as a spontaneous dissection, e.g., in subjects with severe hypertension.

The acute event narrows or completely obliterates the carotid lumen, blocking the flow to the brain. Sudden, severe cerebral symptoms, often acute neck pain, and a localized tenderness at the mandibular angle may indicate this condition. Arteriography shows a "tapered" narrowing of the carotid; the distal lumen may be obliterated and thrombosis may be present.

Anticoagulants are considered the main management method. Intramural clots may be lysed. Stenting (or surgery) may be an indication in patients with recurrent TIAs or severe neurological deficits. Ligation of the carotid can be performed — particularly in younger subjects with good collateral arteries and when the carotid back pressure is >65 mmHg.

Fibromuscular dysplasia

Fibromuscular dysplasia is considered a nonatheroslerotic condition, often affecting young women and usually bilateral. The primary lesion caused by an increase in fibrotic components of the arterial wall with overgrowth of the media has a segmental distribution causing irregular narrowing of the arteries.

A series of apparent, concentric rings are seen as the most common lesions with a radiological appearance of a string of beads along the arteries including the internal carotid. About 30% of these patients may be hypertensive for a renal artery stenosis. TIAs and stroke may also be observed in some 20% of these patients. Interventional correction — by angioplasty or surgery with dilatation or substitution of the stenosed segments may have good results.

10

Renovascular Hypertension

Introduction

Less than 3% of hypertensive patients with a difficult control of blood pressure may have a renovascular disease. The condition is mostly athero-sclerotic or may be associated to fibromuscular dysplasia (FMD), renal embolization (and even dissection of the renal artery), hypoplasia of the artery, aneurysms, stenosis of the suprarenal aorta causing flow reduction to the kidney.

Atherosclerosis — generally in older patients — produces stenosis at the origin of the main renal artery from the aorta. The severely hypoper-fused kidney is generally smaller. Less frequently, arterial lesions may be present at distal branches inside the kidney. Bilateral lesions are observed in 95% of cases.

FMD tends to involve the middle and distal third part of the main renal artery and it may extend to branches. Medial fibrodysplasia is con-sidered the most common variety of FMD; the disease tends to be bilateral in 50% of these patients. The concentric, sequential rings of hyperplasia project into the arterial lumen, causing stenosis. Renal artery aneurysm may coexist.

FMD may affect more frequently young women with an onset of the hypertension before the age of 45. In 10% of children with hypertension, renovascular disease is a possible causative disorder. Developmental renal artery hypoplasia, aortic coarctation and Takayasu arteritis are other clinical conditions causing hypertension in children.

Renal artery stenosis reduces the distal kidney tissue flow. The cells of the juxtaglomerular complex secrete renin which acts on circulating angiotensinogen to form angiotensin I that is rapidly converted into angiotensin II by angiotensin-converting enzyme (ACE). This octapeptide constricts the arterioles, increases aldosterone secretion and promotes sodium retention. Due to the excess in aldosterone, hypertension becomes volume dependent. Over time, morphological changes develop in the kidney structure and hypertension become less sensitive to ACE inhibition.

With sodium restriction and volume reduction (e.g., by diuretics), the hypertension may become once again sensitive to ACE inhibition. If both kidneys have a significant renal artery stenosis, renal insufficiency may occur earlier in the evolution of the disease.

Clinical observations

Subjects are mostly asymptomatic but headache, symptoms of depression in some patients, a persistent elevation of the diastolic pressure may be the only abnormal findings. A renal artery bruit is uncommon; other plaque or intima–media thickening at the carotid, femoral artery and at aortic level may identify the presence of atherosclerosis.

Absence of family history for hypertension and a very early onset (e.g., childhood, early adulthood) may be important indications of renovascular hypertension. Fast progression of hypertension, the resistance to control with antihypertensives are also suggestive of renovascular disease. The rapid deterioration of the renal function may indicate severe renal hypoperfusion.

Renovascular hypertension is suspected when diastolic pressure is constantly high and not easily controllable (e.g., >115 mmHg) and when renal function deteriorates when patients use ACE inhibitors. Sudden onset of pulmonary edema with severe hypertension is also highly suggestive of renovascular hypertension.

Diagnostics

Urinary excretion studies, selective renin determination from renal vein samples, renal scintigraphy and ultrasound may define the clinical picture.

Vascular imaging of the renal arteries is justified in patients who have precipitous drop of blood pressure or/and decreased renal function with ACE, when it is difficult to control hypertension and in all cases of unexplained deterioration in renal function. Contrast in the kidney under unphysiological conditions may further deteriorate renal functions.

Duplex ultrasound screening

Renal artery stenosis (with peak systolic velocity >180 cm/s may suggest stenosis and renal hypoperfusion. Imaging using CTA or MRA may define the arteries more efficiently in this case, but contrast must be used with caution in renal insufficiency. CTA contrast may be nephrotoxic. Gadolinium has been associated with systemic nephrogenic fibrosis in subjects with reduced renal function and clearance.

Renal arteriography is a standard to diagnose stenosis; most often the lesion is at the origin of one of the renal arteries. Imaging of the aorta and renal arteries shows the anatomy of the stenoses. Nonionic contrast agents and hydration are used to prevent renal damage from contrast. N-acetyl cysteine and sodium bicarbonate control a possible tubular necrosis.

Medical management

An aggressive management is needed with control of all risk factors. If hypertension responds to medical therapy and renal function is normal, there is no need for interventional treatments. PGE1 infusion may improve kidney perfusion and may help to reduce the need for other antihypertensive treatments.

Angioplasty has been successfully used but some long-term results have been controversial. Medical management with angiotensin receptor blockers may be effective as stenting in many cases. The need for individual management is important in this condition. Fibromuscular dysplasia appears to respond better to angioplasty.

Surgery (often possible after unsatisfactory angioplasty) must consider the presence of other lesions. Nephrectomy, endarterectomy, bypass, hepatorenal or splenorenal procedures are possible; nonanatomic, auto-transplant of the kidney after extracorporeal correction — on table — of the arterial lesions may be possible solutions to be individualized. Celiac and splenic arteries may also have lesions in subjects with diffuse atherosclerosis.

Prognosis

It is possible to lower blood pressure in 90% of subjects with fibromuscular dysplasia but in segmental, severe atherosclerotic lesions (subjects are generally older), the success rate can be around 60%. Angioplasty and stenting — in great evolution at the moment — may give mixed results and may be associated to microembolization.

11

Mesenteric and Intestinal Ischemia

Introduction

The celiac axis, the superior and inferior mesenteric artery are the most important suppliers to the gut. The internal iliac artery supplies flow to the distal colon. There are many vascular interconnections and most obstructions are, usually, well tolerated as collateral flow is available.

Atheromas cause the most obstructive lesions often at the level of the aortic emergence. Associated plaques are present, usually, in other arteries. Relatively rare is the occurrence of lesions linked to vasculitis, lupus erythematosus, Takayasu (very low frequency). Chronic mesenteric ischemia is characterized by postprandial abdominal pain, abdominal or visceral "angina" starting minutes after eating and lasting from minutes to hours.

Abdominal pain may be severe, localized at the deep epigastrium and radiating laterally. In some patients, this type of pain may mimic angina and MIs. Weight loss may be frequent and malabsorption common. Diarrhea and vomiting are less frequent. Bruits may be present in a few subjects in defined positions.

Diagnostic

Ultrasound may be diagnostic in typical cases or can be used in most cases as a screening to image the mesenteric arteries and the celiac axis. The scanning of patients is more effective when the subject is standing.

CTA or specific mesenteric angiography is needed for a specific diagnosis; lateral projections show the arteries. Some angiograms may produce mesenteric artery thrombosis. Hydration is therefore determinant after angio.

Treatment

Direct, surgical correction, percutaneous transluminal angioplasty (PTA) and stenting are possible in most cases. Single, focal lesions may be treated with the best results. Embolization and thrombosis may happen during these procedures. Surgical revascularization, with endarterectomy, and patch or graft replacement have been successfully used.

A retroperitoneal approach is often possible. All aortic lesions should also be considered if any interventional treatment may be more difficult in acute vasculitis (these patients may benefit from high doses of steroids and immunosuppressive agents). Improving perfusion with PGE1 infusions gives immediate benefits but the effects are temporary.

Prognosis

The relief of symptoms may be obtained in most patients. Endovascular treatment may be not durable but all these methods are in evolution.

Acute mesenteric ischemia

Acute mesenteric ischemia is characterized by high mortality rate. Severe, uncontrollable, diffuse abdominal pain without other physical findings (abdominal tenderness or distension) is usually observed. Unless there is a necrosis or a perforation with an acute abdomen, the clinical picture may be difficult to understand.

The onset is generally acute in embolism or in thrombotic occlusion of the superior mesenteric artery. Some symptoms associated to mesenteric ischemia may be present before the crisis. The diagnosis is generally difficult and delays may cause bowel ischemia.

If loop necrosis occurs and bowel resections are needed, the mortality tends to be high. Prognosis: clinical results improve if a good revascularization can be obtained before any intestinal infarction occurs. This requires an early diagnosis that is often only clinical — and complex — in most patients.

12

Celiac Artery Compression and Arterial Aneurysms

Celiac artery compression (median arcuate ligament syndrome)

This condition is a rare cause of intestinal ischemia affecting young adults, mainly women. An epigastric bruit may be present in defined positions. Weight loss is considered common. The diaphragm compresses the artery which may appear scarred and irregular.

Treatment

Reparation of the anatomy with release of the compressing ligament may solve the problem. However, the diagnosis may be difficult and several imaging studies in different positions may be needed.

Surgery — after excluding other problems causing pain — is the most effective solution. Some compression of the celiac artery from the ligament is almost normal but it may disappear with changes in positions. Ultrasound with the patients standing may show the anomaly. Median arcuate ligament compression responds well to surgery but some patients may have limited benefits.

Arterial aneurysms

Aneurysms are localized dilatations of arteries — at least 1.5 times their normal dimension — affecting all vessels. Expanding vessels also tend to elongate in most cases, making the artery tortuous.

A true aneurysm consists of a primary dilatation of the artery including all vessel layers. False aneurysms are caused by a disruption of the arteries without involving all layers of the wall. Often, what looks like an aneurysm is a pulsatile hematoma, not contained by the artery but by an external fibrous, reactive capsule.

False aneurysms caused by infections are often defined mycotic aneurysms even in absence of mycotic positivity. The most common false aneurysms are observed at the femoral artery and are generally a consequence of puncture and catheterization.

Abdominal aortic aneurysms (AAAs) that are infrarenal are the most common conditions involving a true aneurysm. All other arteries may be affected. Iliac, popliteal, aortic arch, descending thoracic aorta (including dilatations after aortic dissection), common femoral artery, carotid artery and the other arteries may develop aneurysms. Rarer causes of aneurysms are conditions like Marfan syndrome, Ehlers–Danlos syndrome, Behçet disease, cystic medial necrosis.

Abdominal aortic aneurysms

The rupture may cause — and used to cause in the recent past — a significant number of deaths in older subjects (aging >65, often with concomitant cardiovascular disease). Easily, some 2% of elderly males, particularly those with significant risk factors, may have an abdominal aneurysm. The incidence of aneurysms and rupture is generally higher in subjects with uncontrolled, higher risk conditions.

The causes of the initial formation of aneurysms and the evolution of these lesions are not completely understood. Atherosclerosis, altered wall perfusion by the vasa vasorum, medial necrosis, increased protease activity, enzymatic destruction of elastin and collagen may all be involved in different cases. Hemodynamic factors (including pressure), irregular pulsatile stress associated to flow into the many branches in the abdominal aorta, a genetically weaker structure of the wall may all contribute.

Experimental studies indicate that the destruction of vasa vasorum in the aorta of animals produces wall dilatations and aneurysms. Diabetics appear to have a lower incidence of AAA. The aortic segment between the renal arteries and the iliac bifurcation includes 90% of all dilatations and the iliac arteries may be included.

Rupture of the sac is the major final event and risk: it is not predictable but the bigger the aneurysm, the higher the risk. Subjects with AAA are generally asymptomatic; ultrasound screening in subjects >65 years (particularly males and or smokers) is very effective and fast.

Even in asymptomatic subjects, an abnormal pulsatility or back pain is not rare. A pulsatile abdominal mass can be felt in most patients (unless obese). An increased tenderness of the mass suggests a clinical evolution (initial or contained dissection). Pain without dissection or rupture is generally associated with local inflammation (the aorta in these cases is surrounded by an inflammatory reaction).

Imaging

Imaging by ultrasound is easy and fast; it can be diagnostic in a matter of minutes; repeated scans evaluate a possible progression in time. These scans may be more difficult in obese patients. CT scans, MRI with 3D reconstruction are diagnostic and useful to plan for invasive procedures. Size determination may be more difficult with tortuosity of the arteries.

CT/MRA both show the precise anatomic location, the presence of wall thrombi, the surrounding anatomy; CT is essential for surgery (the evaluation includes the visualization of horseshoe kidney). Renal abnormalities, venous abnormalities, duplication of the cava may all play a significant role during surgery. With multiplanar CT, angiogram is not indispensable in most cases. However, the peripheral circulation should always be evaluated before surgery.

The natural evolution of aneurysms is now changing with an aggressive control of risk factors. Most dilatations slowly enlarge but some aneurysms may remain stable for a long time without rupture. If a growth rate of 0.5 cm in 6 months is detected, the dilatation is considered in rapid enlargement and some action is suggested.

Over a 5-year period, 40% of AAA of 5.5–6 cm in diameter or larger may be expected to rupture, if left untreated. The average survival of these patients without any management or treatment may be around 16–18 months. When the aneurysms have a diameter of 4–5.4 cm, interventional management is considered and for AAA >5.5 cm, surgery appears to be the best option to avoid complications. Symptomatic (painful) AA or rapidly enlarging dilatations suggest the need for fast action.

Treatment

A synthetic graft, with metal stents is often employed. The aorta proximal to the AAA must have a cylindrical configuration (with a diameter >1.5 cm) to allow adequate sealing.

If the iliac arteries are of sufficient size and have a limited tortuosity, devices can be introduced from the femoral artery. A system of guidewires and specific delivery are used. Endovascular repair exposes patients to low blood loss, meaning that hospital stay may be shorter with an expected reduction in morbidity in comparison with conventional open surgery.

Complications include persistent types of reperfusion of the aneurysm (defined as "endoleaks"). Type 1 endoleak is due to ineffective proximal or distal sealing with pressurization of the AA sac, and this should be fixed immediately. Type 2 endoleak is due to persistent flow through the AA between branches from the inferior mesenteric artery to a patent lumbar artery. These leaks tend to have low pressure and unless the AA is enlarging, the leak is not expected to need immediate treatment. Pressurization of the AA through the graft is defined as a type 3 endoleak. The graft should be repaired or replaced in case of enlargement in subjects with type 2 or 3 endoleaks.

Rupture may also, rarely, occur after endovascular repair. Endograft repair is generally more expensive than open repair. The costs are due to the devices and to the need for closer follow up.

Conventional open repair of AAA consists of replacing the aorta and the bifurcation with a synthetic graft. The proximal anastomosis is made above the aneurysm and distal anastomosis are made on the basis of the extension of the enlargement to the iliac arteries.

Elective management is associated with a 2–4% death rate and with 5–10% of complications. A transperitoneal approach, when possible, can be used instead of a midline laparotomy. The retroperitoneal approach may decrease the incidence of gastrointestinal and pulmonary complications.

In some of these patients, tumors may be concomitant but the repair of the AA is considered the first procedure to perform. Survival is largely determined by any atherosclerotic coronary involvement or by the presence of heart failure and pulmonary problems.

Complications

Bleeding, MI, peripheral ischemia, embolization, spinal ischemia can be controlled in most patients. A contained rupture causes free but limited bleeding into the peritoneal cavity.

Rupture

The interval between the first bleeding due to rupture and a possible death from bleeding is determinant. Bleeding can be controlled with aggressive management but it may also be spontaneously contained by retroperitoneal tissues.

Sudden abdominal pain, radiating to the back or to the inguinal region may be a sign of contained rupture. Blood loss — if important — produces syncope. After a first, initial hemorrhage, pain and lower pressure may decrease the rate of bleeding. A pulsatile abdominal mass, painful, with a picture of an acute abdomen may rise suspicion of contained rupture.

In case of even slight suspicion, an ultrasound scan soon shows the AA and may show the bleeding. Aggravating shock, hypotension and even anuria may follow this in a certain time frame. CT scans are in most cases fully diagnostic, if there is time. Often, however, the surgeon has no time: ultrasound is good enough to proceed to surgery. AA associated with an acute abdomen should go to surgery as soon as possible to control bleeding. Often, revitalizing patients, e.g., with fluids or transfusions, may again increase the bleeding controlled by lower pressures. The surgical control of the aorta proximal and distal is always a priority.

Mortality after rupture is generally due to the general conditions of these patients, to management and to the fast control of bleeding. Still, the death rate can be high and it is generally dependent upon the global management of the problem (not only the surgery). Without surgery, however, rupture is almost always fatal. Some cases of rupture, depending upon conditions and time of arrival to the managing center, can be treated with endovascular stent graft. A complication of surgery for rupture may be retroperitoneal hematoma.

13

Iliac Aneurysms

Introduction

Enlargements of the iliac artery are considered aneurysmatic when they are greater in diameter than the aortic diameter, up to 4 cm. These aneurysms may be asymptomatic for long periods or cause some compression with obstruction of the ureters or neuropathy. Leg swelling may indicate compression of the vein or a deep vein thrombosis (DVT).

Iliac dilatations are often concomitant to AAA and are considered rare as single, localized dilatations. When the enlargement is >3.5 cm, the lesion needs an aggressive follow up even when asymptomatic. With a dilatation >4 cm, repair must be considered.

Management: CT scans, MRI and angio are usually diagnostic. Ultrasound may be difficult at pelvic level. An abdominal or transperitoneal approach to the iliac arteries is defined according to individual conditions. The presence of associated, possible peripheral ischemia should be considered. Any surgery must be planned to preserve pelvic flow into at least one internal pelvic artery. Erectile dysfunction and buttock claudication may occur after surgery.

Suprarenal aortic aneurysms

Around 10% of the AAAs may be suprarenal and approximately 6% may be pararenal. This type of lesion requires a more complex treatment that may have higher risks.

The involvement of the renal arteries may double the operative mortality with renal failure more common after surgery. Revascularization of the celiac axis may also be needed in some patients and methods to preserve the kidneys (intra-arterial perfusion) are often needed.

A left heart bypass is used in true thoracoabdominal AA. Endovascular repair using branched systems has improved survival producing a lower mortality rate but it may be technically difficult in many patients. In higher-risk subjects, branched graft repair tends to be comparable to the best reports for open repair. Kidney autotransplant may be needed.

Inflammatory aneurysms

Degenerative aneurysms with a strong inflammatory response of the surrounding tissues are usually difficult to manage. Retroperitoneal fibrosis may be confined to the anterior aorta and to the iliac arteries. Spontaneous pain and tenderness to palpation may be present. Ureteral obstruction may be present in some 25% of these patients.

Imaging studies (CT scans and MRI) confirm the diagnosis. Medical treatment before surgery may be needed to decrease the level of inflammation. The inflammation tends to disappear or decrease after a successful repair. Recently, endovascular repair has been considered more effective than standard, open surgery for these patients in most cases.

Popliteal and peripheral aneurysms

These lesions are generally silent, often bilateral or cause compression problems and DVT. They become symptomatic when they cause repeated embolization and eventually ischemia. Muscular or ligament compression of the arterial wall may be associated to the genesis of the aneurysmal sac.

Ultrasound is generally easily diagnostic considering that all these aneurysms are relatively superficial. CTA or MRI before surgery defines anatomy and possible compressions and must show the distal peripheral circulation. Thrombolysis is considered disappointing.

Surgical repair is considered essential when the sac has a diameter >2 cm or when the dilatations include thrombi that may embolize (or after embolization). Also, surgery is important when compression may cause symptoms. Peripheral ischemia, if concomitant, requires specific management.

Pseudoaneurysms after catheterization

Bleeding, thrombosis and embolization are the most important complications of these lesions following invasive procedures. When the dilatation of the arterial segment is greater than 2 cm, surgery may be essential. Early surgery when the lesion is <2 cm is indicated in the case of peripheral embolization, mural thrombosis or peripheral ischemia.

Ultrasound is not always conclusive. CT, MRI and angio may also be needed to evaluate the distal arteries. Bypass with a saphenous vein — with exclusion or resection of the affected segment — is the most frequent solution. Endovascular repair may be possible but is considered less durable. Some pseudoaneurysms may be noninvasively treated with ultrasound-guided compression and thrombin injection if the lesions are small and peripheral flow is adequate.

Infected or mycotic aneurysms

These lesions are rarely fungal and their origin may be complex. Microbial aortitis, bacterial contamination of the aortic wall, *Salmonella* infections are the most frequent forms of bacterial contamination. *Staphylococcus* infection after intravenous drugs have been shown. Aortic infection may be the predominant infection.

These lesions include rapidly enlarging aneurysms with general and local signs of infections. Urethral obstruction may be associated. CT scans show the lesions and the inflammatory tissue. The infiltration of the aortic wall is recognized during surgery. Dense inflammatory tissue with fibrotic or partially necrotic material may include the duodenum, the left renal vein, the inferior vena cava (IVC) and any structure close to the aorta. Angiography may show the presence of false aneurysms.

At the moment, an endovascular repair is the best option — when possible — in most patients. Open surgery with excision of the inflamed segment and bypass is also effective but may be complex and may damage organs close to the aorta. Muscle flaps have been used to cover the inflamed arterial segments making healing safer and faster. Antibiotics are considered essential. Generally, there is a regression of the local infection after a successful repair. The long-term patency of the aorta tends to be good.

Radial artery false aneurysms

These lesions are most common with the diffuse use of the artery for catheters. In some aneurysms, infections are present. Imaging shows patency of the collateral flow. Repair is by excision or ligation of the artery with vein segment replacement when the collateral flow is not adequate.

The ulnar collateral flow must be considered before a possible repair. Distal vascular lesions may be diagnosed with ultrasound but the final evaluation — to plan a surgical reconstruction — requires angiography. Distal, palmar small aneurysms may be caused by repetitive trauma and cause embolization or ischemia.

Splenic artery aneurysms

These lesions are generally single lesions occurring in young subjects and are considered a malformation. They are more common in women and may be associated to fibrodysplasia; in some cases, portal hypertension may be associated. These aneurysms tend to be asymptomatic in most cases and are difficult to detect.

A rupture is considered uncommon (<2%) in all splenic aneurysms and the risk of rupture increases when the diameter of the artery is >2–3 cm. There is a connection with pregnancy, particularly in the third trimester: a rupture is associated to severe prognosis with some 75% of maternal deaths and some 90% of fetal deaths.

The diagnosis may occur during a screening with ultrasound; scans with ultrasound may show calcifications at the upper, left quadrant close to the spleen. In these cases, surgery/intervention — as soon as possible in pregnant women — may solve the problem. In low risk subjects with lesions smaller than >3 cm, an endovascular solution is possible but on an individual basis. Laparoscopic ligation of the artery with splenectomy is also a possible solution.

Hepatic artery aneurysms

These appear to be more frequent in men and may have a risk of rupture around 20% with a high mortality rate. Rupture into the biliary tree is possible causing hemobilia. Recurrent abdominal pain and the associated pain + gastrointestinal bleeding + jaundice suggests an intrabiliary rupture. After a full scan of the liver and the spleen with a full angiographic evaluation (when possible), the bleeding may be controlled by invasive methods including open surgery. The common hepatic artery can be ligated if the collateral flow via the gastroduodenal artery is sufficient. A vascular reconstruction may be possible in some cases. Endovascular procedures are becoming more frequent according to the anatomy of the lesions.

Superior mesentric artery aneurysms

This type of aneurysm involves the origin of the branches and may cause abdominal pain. Occasional ultrasound screening may reveal the lesions. The diagnosis requires a CT angio, possibly showing all possible vascular connections and collaterals.

Surgical ligation is possible when collateral flow is adequate; vascular replacement is less common and graft cannot be used in cases associated with arterial infections. Bowel resections may be required when distal branches are involved. Between 50% and 60% of these aneurysms are considered mycotic or infective and require specific care.

Renal artery aneurysms

Renal artery aneurysms are uncommon; it seems possible that they are slightly frequent in women and are idiopathic, although muscular fibrodysplasia, arteritis and microaneurysms may be associated with these. Hypertension may be related to an altered, distal hypoperfusion. Proximal, primary or secondary branches of the renal arteries may be involved. Rupture of these aneurysms is considered rare but may occur in pregnant women. Ultrasound can occasionally show these lesions: specific imaging studies and angiography are needed to evaluate the extension and flow in the aneurysms.

Surgery is considered essential in pregnancy and when aneurysms are large and at risk of rupture. *In vivo* vascular repair or *ex vivo* repair of the most important arterial lesion (with autotransplant) is possible while endovascular options — in rapid evolution — may be still limited and based on individual anatomic considerations. Nephrectomy is always an option.

14

Vasoconstriction, Acrocyanosis and Thoracic Outlet Syndrome

Vasoconstriction

Increased activity of the sympathetic nervous system causes persisting vasoconstriction reducing arteriolar and capillary flow and perfusion (both the thermoregulatory and nutritional components). Raynaud's disease and phenomenon is associated to pallor–cyanosis and rubor after exposure to cold or lower temperature. Extremities tend to be equally affected. However, hands and fingers, being more exposed than feet/toes are mostly affected. The vasoconstriction is more visible at the extremities.

Vasoconstriction, increased viscosity, a subsequent reflex vasodilatation produce — in a standard, not always replicable model — a sequence of white–blue–red color changes in the skin. In Raynaud's disease, spasm acts alone and there is no significant arterial lesion: the course of this conditions is generally benign. Sudden progression with persisting hypoperfusion suggests the presence of arterial lesion associating stenosis and vasoconstriction. Some lesions may be associated to connective tissue disorders (scleroderma, lupus) or to treatments used to control these conditions (e.g., interferon).

Drug-induced vasculitis or vasospasm is a different clinical entity. Also, ischemia and vasospasm (in a very reactive vascular territory as the hands) and repeated embolization is a completely different disease.

Angioneurosis arises from nerve/vascular damage due to repeated trauma (e.g., hammers) or cold-induced vasoconstriction and is a completely different condition. Workers digging tunnels in the cold and using vibrating instruments may have this specific angioneurosis that is considered a professional disease. Cold agglutinins, conditions such as chronic renal failure, the presence of tumors and some drugs may suddenly produce vasospasm in subjects that had never observed this problem.

An increased reactivity to cold and cold stimuli is — generally — the initial presentation and often the only problem in patients with vasospasm. Looking for potential causes may be disappointing as patients (generally young women with minimal subcutaneous tissue and longer fingers) are "congenitally" fast–high responders to cold. Avoiding exposure, smoking and some drugs (betablockers, ergotamine) may improve the vasoconstriction. Nifedipine may help some patients.

PGE1 infusion is effective and often diagnostic as the vasospasm is dissolved for days (in subjects with significant symptoms). Ketanserin or cilostazol have been used and have been effective in controlling symptoms in some patients. However, the main problem for vasospastic disorders is the climate. In places where the average temperature remains around zero for months, this condition is frequent and may have important social and medical consequences (e.g., necrosis and infection). Subjects working in refrigerators or with cold are also at risk.

Most cases do not need medicalization but only need to avoid cold and thermal jumps. The role of uric acid may be important in causing comparable symptoms in young patients (chilblains). Progression of symptoms in vasospastic disorders with final tissue loss and even localized gangrene at the fingertips is now uncommon and may be caused by neglect. Repeated PGE1 infusion — in association with preventive measures — will treat all true vasospastic conditions and eventually help in limiting tissue losses and even amputation.

Acrocyanosis

Overlapping Raynaud's syndrome, this condition is considered a benign problem in young women associated to a lasting cyanosis of the extremities. These patients are generally women with long fingers, with limited subcutaneous tissue. Acrocyanosis may also affect feet (usually covered by shoes). The alterations of the hand tend to disappear in a warm environment or may be associated to hyperhidrosis. Legs may show vasoconstricting patterns defined as cutis marmorata or livedo reticularis.

All arterial pulses are normal or may show a mild decrease in pulsatility during the cold phases regaining a normal wave pattern with warming. PGE1 infusions may produce lasting benefits in association with a protective behavior limiting the risk factors causing the problem (including stressing conditions).

Thoracic outlet syndrome (TOS)

Abnormal compression of arterial–venous–nervous paths and brachial plexus proximal to neck may cause problems defined as TOS. Abnormal cervical ribs, an anomalous first rib or ligaments, the hypertrophy of the anterior scalene muscle, or position changes may compress the neurovascular bundle. Irregular healing with hypertrophic bone scars after a fracture may also cause compressions.

Symptoms may arise in adults after full growth and may be transient or associated to positional changes altering flow or compressing the nerve structure. Neurological symptoms tend to predominate over the ischemic component. Compression of the subclavian artery when severe may be associated to postcompression dilatation which may cause distal embolization.

Venous compression may cause thrombosis but rarely the obstruction is severe and the risk of embolization is limited. Exercise of the arm may increase or improve some symptoms. The Pager–Schroetter syndrome is a compression associated with exercise-related symptoms causing thrombosis. Neurological symptoms are predominant when the brachial plexus is involved with a mainly ulnar distribution.

Symptoms are associated to defined positions (e.g., hyperabduction, traction). Numbness of the affected limb may occur during rest or sleep.

- Electromyography reveals the level of compression and the entity of the neurological damage.

- In persisting cases, muscle atrophy may occur.
- A positive Adson test with weakening of pulses on rotation of the head to the other side is not very diagnostic as it may be present even in normal subjects.
- Digital pressure on the plexus may reproduce symptoms.
- Arterial symptoms are not very common and arterial ischemia is usually due to embolization.
- Venous occlusion is the cause of unilateral arm swelling.
- Neurological tests should exclude other problems (cervical disk).

CT scans or MRI require interpretation and ultrasound may be difficult. The anatomy may change in different positions of the arm. Arteriography whilst changing positions may show a stenosis with arm in abduction. Even an angiogram may be nondiagnostic. The observation of a poststenotic dilatation defines the problem.

Management

- Postural changes may be very effective in some patients.
- Medical treatment has minimal value and is used as a palliative and when surgery is not possible.
- In young, active patients, surgery is the best option, with specific decompression particularly when a strong neurological component and atrophy are present.
- The resection of an abnormal first rib may be resolutive.
- The supraclavicular approach may be difficult in some patients.
- Irregular anterior scalene muscles and any abnormal fibrous band may be resected.
- An arterial stenosis requires decompression with arterial reconstruction.
- If edema is severe, venous thrombosis can be treated with catheter-direct thrombolysis before attempting surgical decompression.
- These lesions have a good prognosis in otherwise healthy patients.

15

Arteriovenous Fistulas

Introduction

Arteriovenous (AV) fistulas are malformations (congenital or acquired) in which the arterial flow goes into the venous circulation without a passage in the capillary system. The lesions are very variable in anatomy and may have a significant systemic effect. Multiple small communications may increase venous return, cause organ hypertrophy, swelling, the arterialization of veins (that become pulsatile). The systemic involvement is shown by the increased heart rate eventually leading — when flow is high — to an increase in ventricular size and even heart failure.

Acquired, posttraumatic or postsurgical AV communications can produce dramatic clinical pictures and heart failure may occur rapidly. AV communications in the gastrointestinal tract may cause bleeding difficult to identify. The rare Osler–Weber–Rendu syndrome (hereditary hemorrhagic telangiectasia) is associated to intestinal bleeding and epistaxis caused by large arteriovenous malformations in the GI tract and in the lungs. Lung vascular lesions recirculate blood with lower pO_2 causing finger clubbing, cyanosis and polycythemia.

The fistulas created for hemodialysis constitute a completely different pathophysiological condition. Acquired fistulas due to trauma, punctures, catheters, erosion of aneurysm into a vein also cause acute communication with severe, dramatic consequences — according to the shifted volume — if untreated. There are reports of aortic aneurysms rupturing into the cava. In these patients, cardiac dilatation and failure may occur in a short time.

Clinical observations

A murmur, a palpable thrill, vein dilatation with pulses and altered high-velocity arterial flow in veins are common. Tachycardia due to increased cardiac load may be a late sign. Pulsations in veins decrease when the fistula is compressed or excluded. CT scans or MRI shows the extent of the communications and the tissue involvement. CT angio shows the communication channels but the imaging is generally difficult as several communications may be involved.

Treatment

There is no standard management. Conservative progressive treatment — e.g., compression — may have some effects and avoid some complications (e.g., the asymmetrical growth of a limb) but are difficult to achieve.

Often many lesions are inaccessible and surgery can be disappointing. Catheter embolization tends to be successful in limited areas and often needs repeated session. AV communications of the head, neck and pelvis are possibly the best applications for embolization.

Sclerosing solutions may produce a temporary reduction in flow in low pressure channels (veins) but the communications tend to recur. Surgery may include ligation of some arterial segments but it is very individual — as all lesions are different — and often not resolutive. Covered stents have been used for traumatic fistulas. Treatment is oriented by the specific lesions on an individual basis.

Prognosis

The management is based more on control than on the healing/closure of the communications. Traumatic AV fistulas have better results than congenital lesions. Micro diffuse AV communications are generally very difficult to manage. When a congenital AV malformation is observed, it is better to look for other possible less visible malformations (e.g., at spinal or cerebral level) that may coexist and modify the prognosis.

Arteriovenous fistula for hemodialysis

A fistula with good flow requires a large vein (<5 mm) superficial enough for some 20 cm. The cephalic vein is considered adequate. A vein may dilate from 3.4 to 5–6 mm after arterialization.

The connection of the radial artery to the cephalic vein creates an AV communication good for hemodialysis. A prosthetic graft can be used if veins are not available but the survival of these loops are some 40% at 2 years with higher risks for infections.

All veins need to arterialize before being used for cannulation. This process requires about 6 weeks. The flow rate for an efficient dialysis should be around 300 mL/min. Arteriovenous accesses should be watched very carefully for arterial steal and distal ischemia, particularly in diabetics. Bleeding from an access may be lethal.

The Venous System

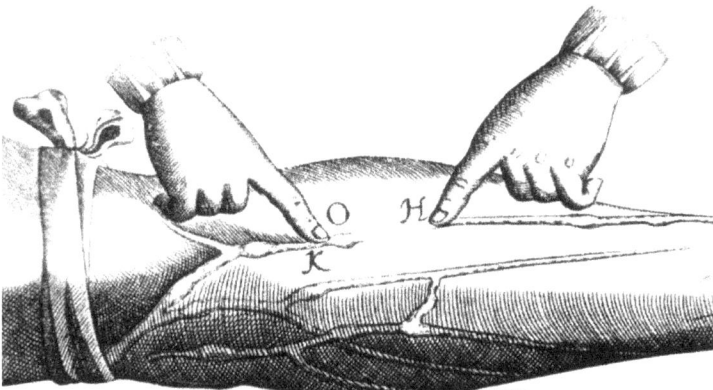

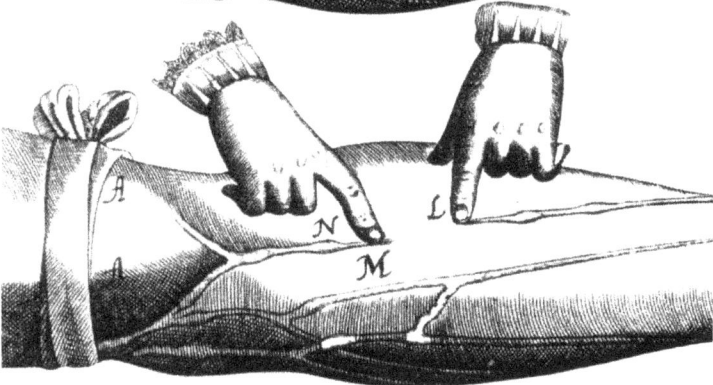

16

Varicose Veins

Introduction

Varicose veins (VV) is a condition which knows no social boundary. Untreated VV is linked to chronic venous hypertension in all strata of society and across all genders; it is a cause of chronic venous insufficiency (CVI) from which untreated VV will produce capillary and skin alterations, pigmentations and venous hypertensive microangiopathy.

This condition when untreated may eventually cause venous ulcerations leading to severe disability, with high personal and social costs. Due to the wide remit of the condition, the problem of VV has been schematically subdivided into primary and secondary categories.

Real or primary VV can be prominent and irregular in caliber, often dysanatomical with normal segments and enlargements and a serpiginous more than a rectilinear course. Secondary veins are usually associated with the consequences of DVT, AV communications, compression of proximal vein trunks increasing distal pressure and pregnancy (in which case most veins may disappear after the end of pregnancy). Dilated veins keep their shape; they appear larger and prominent.

Etiologic factors and distribution

No clear factors — that may be eventually controlled or corrected — have been identified in the development of VV; this multicausal abnormality and clinical condition may evolve into medical problems.

VV are asymptomatic in many subjects for many years. Pain, swelling, edema develop in time with CVI and assume clinical relevance according to individual characteristics and habits; progressive skin pigmentation is associated to long-term presence of CVI.

When veins are prominent, dilated and varicose, superficial thrombosis even from minimal trauma may develop and significant bleeding may occur even with a minor cut. These signs — thrombosis and bleeding — are considered the classic indication for surgical treatment.

Clinical evaluation of the veins (with the patient standing) does not give a complete clinical picture. Inspection may be difficult and misleading. Thermography helps to localize in seconds the most prominent veins (even those that are difficult to see are easily detected by thermography). The presence of thrombotic or inflamed segments is revealed in real time and becomes a target for investigation.

Signs associated with VV and CVI tend to improve with rest, legs elevation and effective elastic compression. Several venous products — mostly of natural origin — effectively control edema and signs/symptoms associated to VV and CVI but have a limited activity of the evolution of the veins and the development of new incompetent segments. These products, usually supplements in pharmaceutical standards (PS supplements), have been evaluated in several studies and appear effective even on the prevention of ulcerations as they control edema.

Most VV are present along the course of the long saphenous vein (LSV) but some veins can be completely separated from the main venous trunks (e.g., linked to a perforating vein). Small reticular veins and telangiectasia may be considered a different disease — more visible when the skin is very transparent — that requires a different, specific management.

Secondary varicose veins — e.g., following an episode of venous thrombosis or a compression — may be associated to CVI and require a comparable evaluation (usually more complex) and management. Thermographic examples of VV are shown in Fig. 1. Ultrasound Duplex is the primary test to show the localization of reflux in the venous network. The test must exclude arterial problems, thrombosis, venous compressions and deep venous problems (e.g., postthrombotic incompetence).

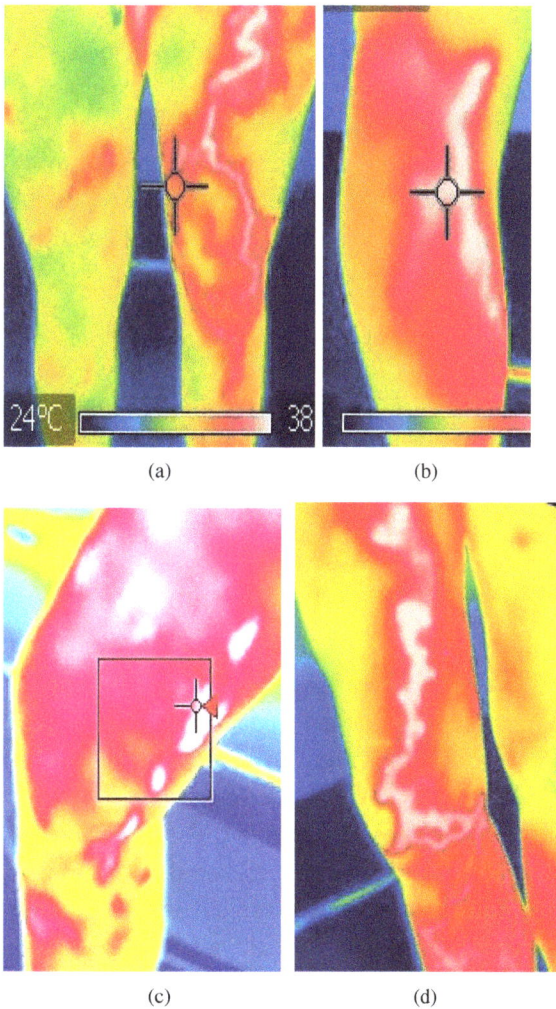

(a) (b)

(c) (d)

Figure 1. Patterns of varicosities are revealed and documented in seconds with ultrafast thermography. The increased temperature in some segment may correspond to local thrombosis and may selectively indicate the target for ultrasound assessment. Images also have a medicolegal value, i.e., before and after treatment. Some veins, difficult to see, are clearly shown on thermography.

The evaluation of the superficial venous system must detect the selective competence of the main junctions at first (saphenofemoral junction (SFJ), popliteal — short saphenous vein junction), major, important venous reflux (e.g., longer than 3 s) and minor points of incompetence. Major (high reflow) and minor reflux (lower reflow, reflux lasting <3 s) points can be identified and considered as significant targets for surgery (or sclerotherapy).

The ultrasound evaluation is simple but the anatomy is different from the more regular anatomy of the arteries and requires some experience. Ideally the surgeon treating the veins should test the patient before management.

Treatments

In brief, the treatment of VV is based on finding the major points of incompetence after excluding DVT and deep venous obstruction.

Conservative management

Compression

Elastic stockings below knee are very effective: stockings — with some 25–35 mmHg of compression at the ankle — can be effective in controlling most symptoms and edema. Climatic conditions may alter compliance. Exercise, leg elevation, avoiding the same positions and constricting clothes, weight control may all help in controlling CVI and its consequences.

Increased venous pressure (e.g., due to deep venous incompetence or obstruction) requires higher pressure stocking that tends to decrease compliance. Strong compression stockings take time to wear and cannot withstand heat.

Sclerotherapy

Sclerotherapy can be used in most patients with smaller veins and no major points of incompetence, as the first option. It may also be used as the main option in most patients when surgery is not possible. Also, it is a good, minimally invasive solution for older patients. Smaller veins (caliber <2 mm) and vein segments may be controlled exclusively with sclerotherapy with good, long-term results.

Below-knee veins respond much better to sclerotherapy and compression. Also, vein segments not directly connected with the LSV or other main trunks with higher venous pressure and reflux have, generally, good results with sclerotherapy alone.

Surgery

Stripping may be now considered obsolete: often, most of the veins are only dilated and not incompetent. Resolving incompetence — e.g., at the SFJ — may make most of the remaining veins competent. When ligating the SFJ, it is important to avoid thrombosis of the venous segment close to the ligature of the LSV.

Major points of incompetence, when the diameter of the vein is >2–3 mm, with long reflux (e.g., 3 s with duplex on distal compression-release maneuver) should be treated with surgery when possible. Major points of incompetence also have a hemodynamic value and alter ambulatory venous pressure (AVP) and refilling time (RT) making it much shorter. However, all dilated, prominent or visible veins tend to be associated to incompetence and should be destined to management.

Anatomic veins are easier to identify and classify. Often, nonanatomic veins are present for different causes (e.g., in postthrombotic patients, after previous surgery). These veins should be singularly evaluated and their major incompetence levels (the origin of the reflux) should be identified.

The association of superficial and deep venous incompetence is common. As the possibilities of management for the deep venous system are still limited, the surgeon must aggressively focus on what can be managed in the superficial system. Even a minimal increase in venous pressure (e.g., due to a superficial incompetent segment) may be enough to increase venous pressure and to trigger ulcerations.

Reconstructive attempts have been made to restore superficial competence. The correction of the most common incompetent site, the SFJ, with a specific external venous valve (EVS, Gore, including a nitinol frame in a Gore-Tex flexible structure) may restore competence in the LSV — in selected subjects — with good results after 10 and 20 years. However,

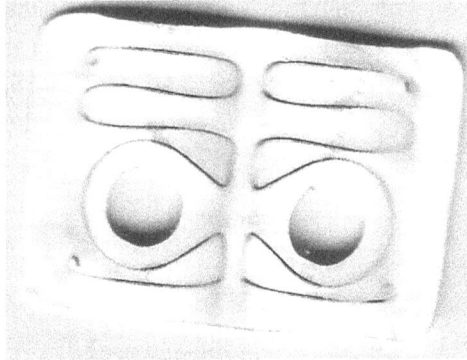

Figure 2.   An external valve system (EVS) developed by Gore in Flagstaff, USA, and implanted by us for the first time may keep the vein competent at the SFJ for years. Selected patients may have benefit. The system was particularly useful to study in time (20 years) selective incompetence of venous segments and how this incompetence may propagate to other venous segments. The SFJ is the natural target for this system that — like many other reconstructive methods — was and is limited to a few centers and did not become a common procedure. Costs were relatively high in comparison with ligation or stripping. The Gore-Tex structure includes a nitinol frame that keeps the "memory" of the intended shape of the vein after the implant.

other incompetence points or VV tend to appear as the natural evolution of VV is difficult to slow down (see Fig. 2).

Conclusions on VV therapies

In summary — ideally — the best options for VV are the following:

(a) the surgical treatment (ligation) of the points of major incompetence (particularly proximal to the knee) in association with
(b) sclerotherapy of below-knee veins.

Solutions must be always individualized and applied according to the social context. In many countries, VV surgery is not reimbursed by healthcare providers as it is not considered life threatening. It must be stressed that all methods to control VV are effective in different ways in good hands. When properly and physiologically used, all methods have good, long-term results. The skill of the operators is more important than the type of treatment.

Surgical and management tips for VV

1. Find all dilated and VV by inspection + thermography.
2. The most visible, prominent veins (and all frankly VV) need management.
3. Define the presence of superficial and/or deep incompetence.
4. Exclude postthrombotic problems (by history, ultrasound) and thrombotic risks.
5. With ultrasound, define the following:
   (a) patency
   (b) deep competence/incompetence
   (c) major incompetence points:
      — SFJ (Figs. 3(a)–3(c))
      — junction of the short saphenous vein
      — perforating veins.
6. Define strategy.
7. Treat major points of incompetence first and from the most proximal (first) to the most distal.
8. Above-knee VV have better results with surgery.
9. Below-knee VV: good effects of sclerotherapy.
10. For younger subjects, the best option is surgery (with better long-term results).
11. For older patients, sclerotherapy is a good option (long-term results are less satisfactory).
12. Sclerotherapy can be repeated if needed.
13. Stripping (Fig. 4), generally, is not needed; the important steps are to eliminate/exclude the incompetence points and segments.
14. Dilated veins may recover their original size when incompetence is corrected.
15. Cost is essential considering the large number of patients.
16. There is no single-event treatment.
17. Most subjects require repeated treatments in time.
18. The best solution for cost efficacy is to use small cuts for major points of incompetence; wait and treat residual veins with sclerotherapy, particularly those below knee.
19. Individual conditions (age, type of activity, etc.) should always be considered.

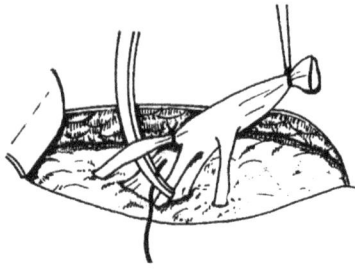

(a)

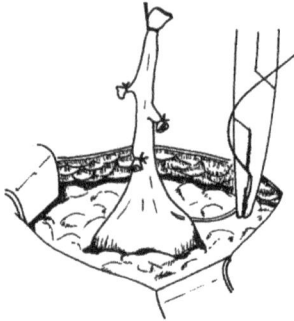

(b)

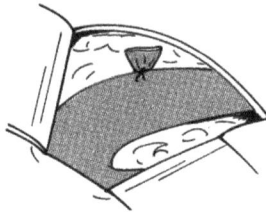

(c)

Figure 3.   Ligation of all collaterals at the SFJ. The size of cuts and the instruments are made bigger in the images to illustrate the concept. Very small cuts and instruments are used now. Collaterals are more frequent in secondary VV. The need to cut all collaterals may be debatable now. Open endothelium in venous stumps may produce revascularization with new vessels around the surgical area. The stump of the saphenous vein should be ligated over a stitch. (a)–(c) Major incompetence points.

(a)

(b)

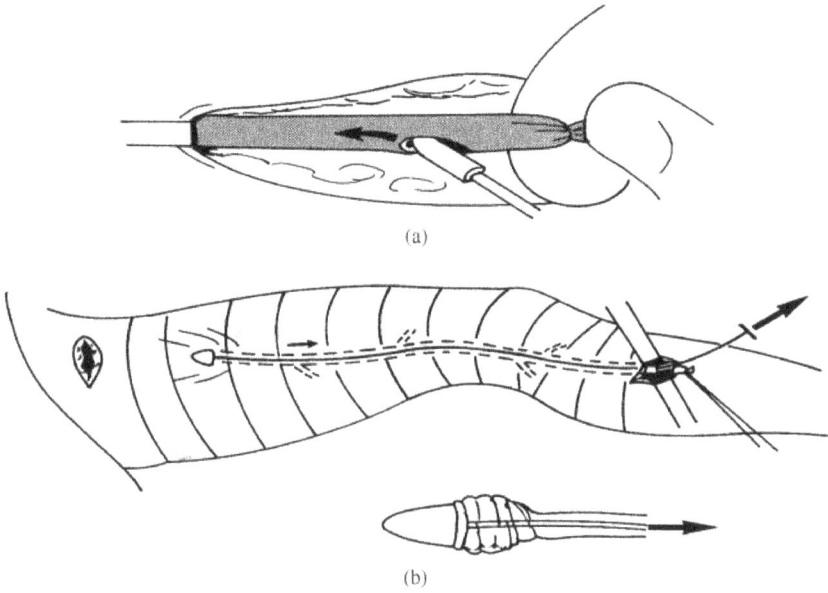

Figure 4.   Stripping with its many evolutions is still used with several variants. This is the classic procedure described by Prof. M. Perrin in the *Encyclopédie Médico-Chirurgicale*. (a) Introduction of the vein stripper into the LSV at the ankle and (b) Stripping.

17

Considering Venous Surgery and Management

Making it simple

Major incompetence at the SFJ can be treated with local anesthetic. Collateral veins at the SFJ should be ligated. In the images, the size of the surgical incision, instruments and needles are exaggerated to make them visible. Actually, very small cuts and needles are used. A good 45% of SFJs have very minimal collaterals.

The SFJ is the most common point of major incompetence in most patients. Even the single ligation of the SFJ may produce a decrease in size of the LSV that may regain competence for years if no other large incompetence points are present. Ligating the LSV and using the residual proximal segment for gentle traction clearly exposes all collaterals. The SFJ without collaterals rarely causes significant incompetence in the future.

Do we really need stripping?

Stripping — still used in some centers — is rarely needed or useful if the points of incompetence are corrected and the main venous segment is made competent. Subjects now arrive to management earlier than years ago when patients arrived to medical observation when the veins were very damaged and dilated (and stripping was justified in many cases).

Using different methods for stripping including heat, radiofrequency nuclear power or dark matter is not always efficient or cost effective; most of the vein can be spared to leave a more physiological, residual venous system.

Treating the short saphenous vein is more difficult from a surgical point of view and the anatomy is more variable. Stripping of the short saphenous vein is not advisable, generally, as it may cause nerve damage and some complications (see Fig. 1).

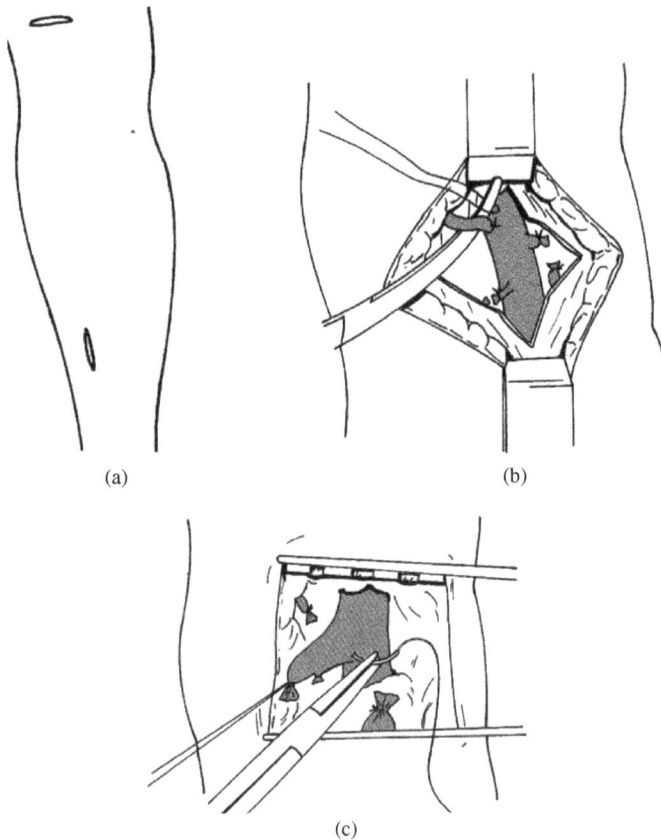

(a)

(b)

(c)

Figure 1.   Ligation or stripping of the short saphenous vein is more anatomically complex and exposes patients to some complications. Compression sclerotherapy as an alternative — when possible — may be very effective below the knee.

Also, all below-knee veins — including posterior veins — may have very good results with sclerotherapy as compression below knee is very effective. A combination of surgery and sclerotherapy is also possible at any level with ligation of the incompetent vein after distal injection of a sclerosing solution. The entire local incompetent distal system can be injected with one single shot. The core business in all vein surgery is to find the incompetent points (the "leaking taps" by ultrasound) and selectively ligate the T-branches.

The T-junction

The T-junction including the vertical branch can be also injected (Fig. 2) and compressed but with less satisfactory long-term results. *This is really the key surgical solution* for most varicose veins (VV) if the skin is surgically accessible (not too thick, ulcerated or inflamed).

The intervention can be repeated several times — similar to that of a dentist's technique — with minimal small cuts and very limited discomfort. It is now more usually associated to sclerotherapy and this combination is the simplest and most cost-effective solution for management. It does not require hospitals and can be done with limited surgical sets (even minimalized disposable sets).

The residual stump at the SFJ

Disconnecting the SFJ and its collaterals (Fig. 3) is the best option to neutralize the biggest, most common leaking point. Big, residual collaterals may dilate and lead to new incompetence. But in some cases, there are minimal collaterals. However, studies show that even a distal ligation at the point where the saphenous vein becomes superficial, some 6 cm below, distal to the SFJ, may completely block incompetence and reflux in most patients.

This more distal cut can be done easily with local anesthetic with a small superficial incision and requires a less advanced skill (and instrumentation) than manipulating the SFJ, close to the femoral vein in a deeper and more complex incision. This technique is more effective in primary VV.

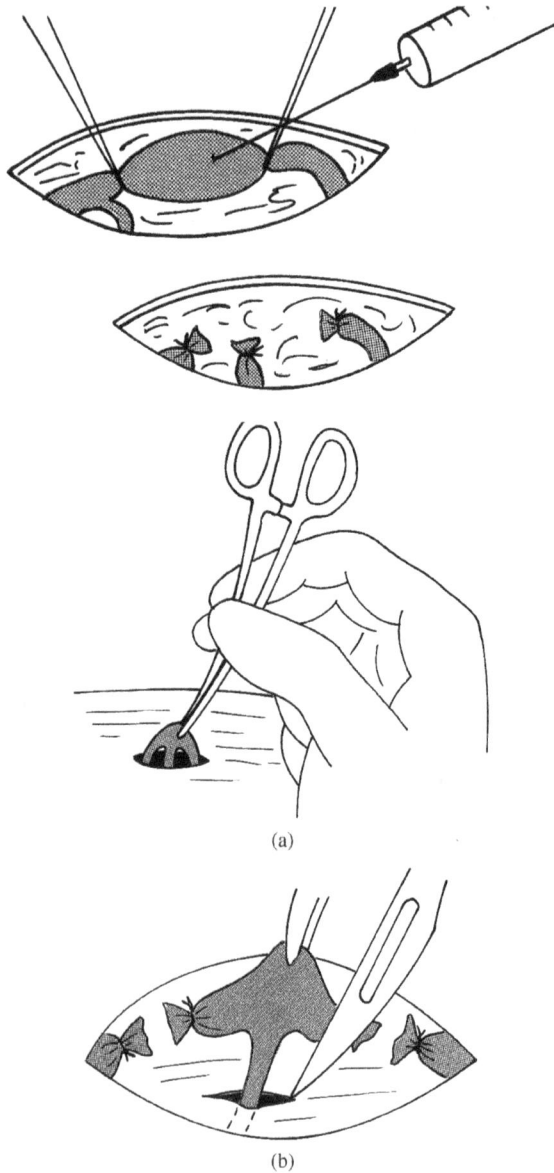

Figure 2.   A combination of surgery and sclerotherapy with injection of the sclerosing agent into the residual vein lumens after ligations may produce better results than simple ligation. (a) Intraoperative, retrograde sclerosing injection of a varicose collateral vein after ligation of the larger varicose trunks and (b) The basis ligation of a T-junction.

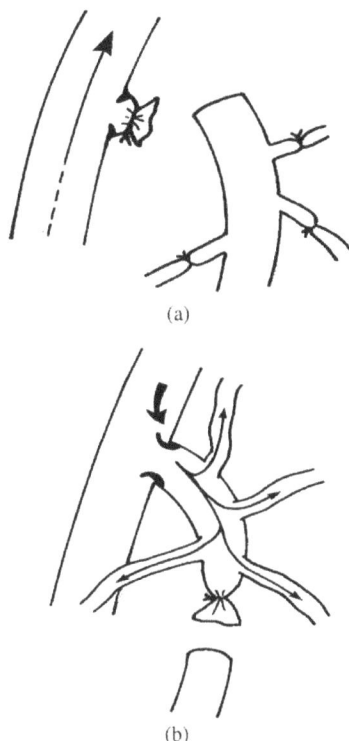

(a)

(b)

Figure 3.   A sample of (a) correct and (b) incorrect ligation at the SFJ, when there are important, hemodynamically relevant collaterals that may expose the superficial venous system to revascularization. This is particularly true in secondary, postthrombotic VV with a long period of increased venous pressure at the common femoral vein level.

Residual vein trunks

After removing the long saphenous vein — if this is the chosen solution — some significant segments may remain anyway and may become more dilated in time (Fig. 4). These segments will probably need management (usually, sclerotherapy is a good solution) after the removal of the main trunk. In 6–12 months, residual incompetent veins may become visible and require a treatment strategy.

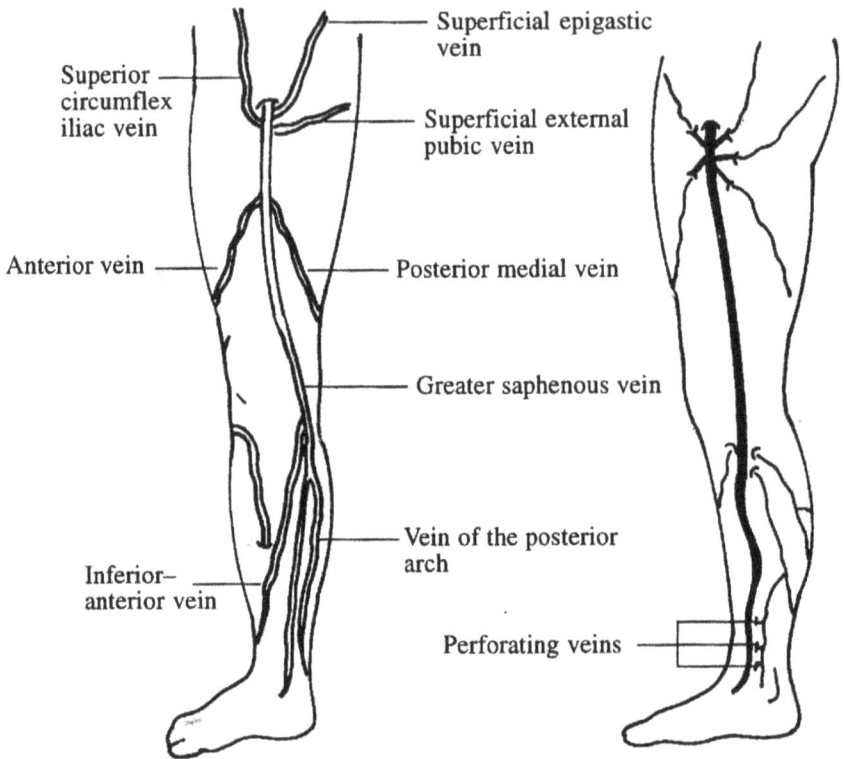

Superficial epigastic vein

Superior circumflex iliac vein

Superficial external pubic vein

Anterior vein

Posterior medial vein

Greater saphenous vein

Vein of the posterior arch

Inferior– anterior vein

Perforating veins

Figure 4. After unselectively removing the LSV, many collaterals may remain and become incompetent in a short period of time creating new important varicosities. This is particularly true for secondary and advanced cases of CVI.

Single incompetence

Some veins are incompetent at their major points of incompetence only (e.g., the SFJ). The dilatation of the vein makes the distal valves incompetent. Blocking incompetence at the SFJ may be enough to make the distal segment competent again (Fig. 5).

Interesting attempts have been made to make the SFJ competent again blocking reflux. A selective external valvuloplasty and a specific external vein valve (Gore) have been used with good results in long-term studies. These methods, however, have not become common as they

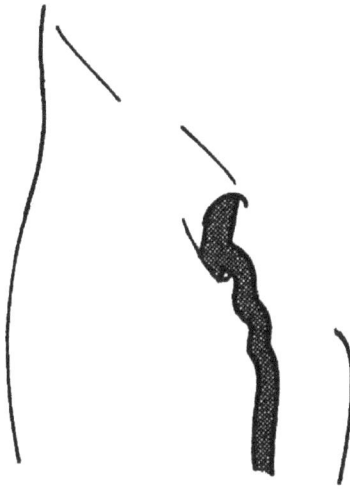

Figure 5. Varicose or dilated? Many veins are just dilated with a major point of incompetence at the SFJ. A very selective ligation of the junction may preserve the vein for many years without the need of removing long segments of vein.

require more skill (valvuloplasty) or higher costs (the external venous valve) and often no patients or providers are interested in paying for a higher level of more physiological surgical attention.

Sclerotherapy

Sclerotherapy is now based on safe injection of a sclerosing fluid into the lumen of a vein. The fluid produces swelling and a strong inflammation of the vein walls. Compression of the vein keeps the two opposing vein walls in contact producing a nonthrombotic closure. The segment eventually becomes atrophic and sclerotic and is excluded from the vein circulation.

This technique is successful in most cases when properly used. It is more useful for small segments of veins than longer segments (e.g., longer than 15 cm). Ideally the most important points of incompetence should be ligated before sclerotherapy to control most of the reflux. In this condition, reflux and venous pressure are reduced and compression is more effective in closing the vein.

The sclerosing agents (sodium tetradecyl sulfate (STD) and aetoxis-clerol are the most used products but several other products are also available) are generally safe and nontoxic at the dosage used for sclero-therapy. Allergic reactions are not common.

- Larger veins (3 mm or more) can be injected with a 3% solution.
- Smaller veins (1–3 mm) can be injected with a 2% solution.
- Very small veins (around 1 mm in caliber) are injected with a 1% solution.
- Minimal veins and telangiectasias are injected with a 0.5% (or lower concentration) solution, or with more diluted solutions and with spe-cific agents for very small veins.

It must be remembered that sclerotherapy, although a simpler method of treatment, is nonetheless *still a surgical method* and should be used *only* by surgeons or physicians with surgical training. In expert hands, side effects are minimal. Repeated sessions, injecting a few veins and compressing a few segments of the legs at the time are cost effective, simple and well tolerated.

The *combination of surgery* (with focus on the *T-branches*) and *scle-rotherapy* at the moment appears to be the simplest and cheapest solution that can be applied to a large number of patients at a low cost, in safety and with minimal alterations in the working life of the patients. The use of foam sclerotherapy is limited to some cases (Fig. 6, popliteal, venous aneurysm, the first reported case). Foam sclerotherapy may cause embolization.

Deep venous incompetence

Deep venous incompetence is generally postthrombotic but may be primary in some patients. The control of reflux within the deep venous system is difficult. It can be achieved with strong compression in most patients. Surgical correction of deep venous incompetence has been attempted successfully in many patients in a few centers. It is not routine.

The incompetent segment (e.g., the popliteal vein) could be replaced in some cases with a segment of vein including one of more valves. However, transplanting a vein segment into a different venous channel

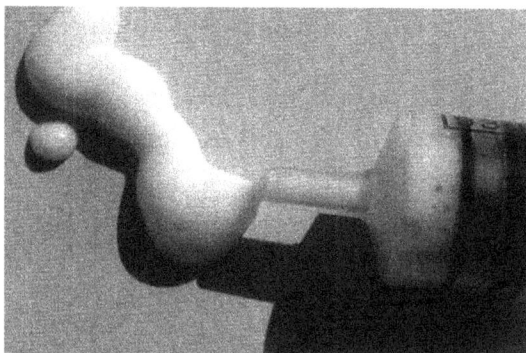

(a)

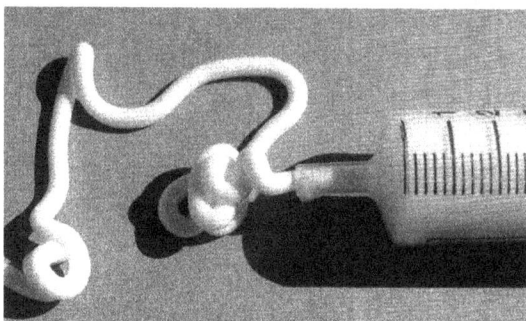

(b)

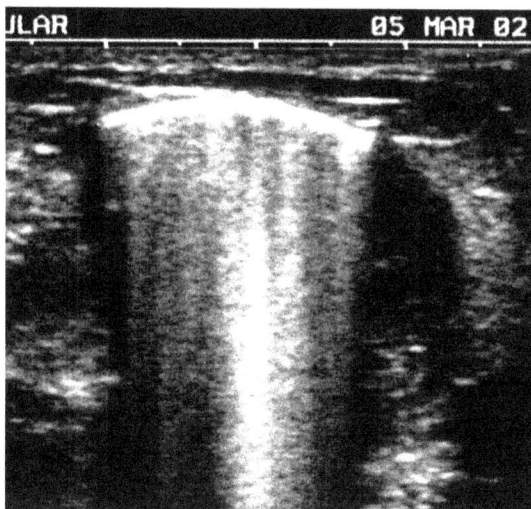

(c)

Figure 6.   Foam sclerotherapy.

(e.g., at the level of the popliteal vein) deprives the transplanted vein of its vasa vasorum.

The transplanted vein segment — without wall perfusion — tends to dilate in time and becomes incompetent. A "net" can be placed around the segment to avoid dilatation.

At the moment, deep venous reconstruction is only for very experienced surgeons in a few centers with specific skills (including the diagnostic part generally based on descending venography).

Klippel–Trénaunay syndrome

Also known as Klippel–Trénaunay–Weber syndrome (angio-osteohypertrophy syndrome, hemangiectasic hypertrophy), Klippel–Trénaunay syndrome (KTS) is a complex condition in which blood vessels and/or lymphatics are badly formed or irregularly connected with the circulation.

KTS is rare; port-wine stains, venous and lymphatic dilatations, hypertrophy and soft tissue thickening are associated. Young subjects may have extensive vein dilatations with atypical venous distribution including anatomical and nonanatomical veins. Arteriovenous communications may increase cardiac output and lead to heart failure. The large veins are exposed to clotting and bleeding.

Treatment is a combination of surgery (debulking, vein ligation, etc.), compression, sclerotherapy and tissue excision and eventually even amputations. It is a very individual disease, often without specific patterns.

Varicose veins during pregnancy

Generally, the prevalent nonanatomical dilatation of veins during pregnancy has a combined origin possibly from hormonal factors and from compression of the iliac veins or cava. Other factors may be involved.

Most veins tend to disappear after pregnancy in 6–12 months; therefore, treatment of residual postpartum veins should be delayed. More veins tend to appear with a new pregnancy.

During pregnancy, compression is important and the best type of antithrombotic prophylaxis should be considered for the most advanced periods.

18

Prevention and Treatment of Venous Thromboembolism

Deep venous thrombosis (DVT)

An abnormal clot in a deep vein (or in an artery) is by definition a thrombus. A clot is a normal condition. A thrombus is always a significant clinical entity. DVT or deep venous thrombosis (usually involving the veins of the legs) is the primary cause of pulmonary thromboembolism (PTE).

Impaired venous return, immobility, stasis, obesity, older age, venous endothelial injury or hypercoagulability have been associated to the genesis of thrombosis. Leg DVT is generally asymptomatic if limited. It may cause leg pain and swelling. The diagnosis is based on history, physical examination (often misleading) and ultrasound; D-dimer is an indication of a thrombotic process but it may be raised by different causes.

The management and treatment of DVTs are based on antico-agulants (particularly when the risk of embolization is higher), compression (stockings) and control of concomitant factors (including immobility). The prognosis is generally good with adequate management. Most DVT episodes in younger — otherwise healthy — subjects (e.g., after a trauma or small fracture) may resolve in weeks without consequences, even without anticoagulants.

Three anatomical types of DVT: (a) distal, (b) proximal and (c) bilateral.

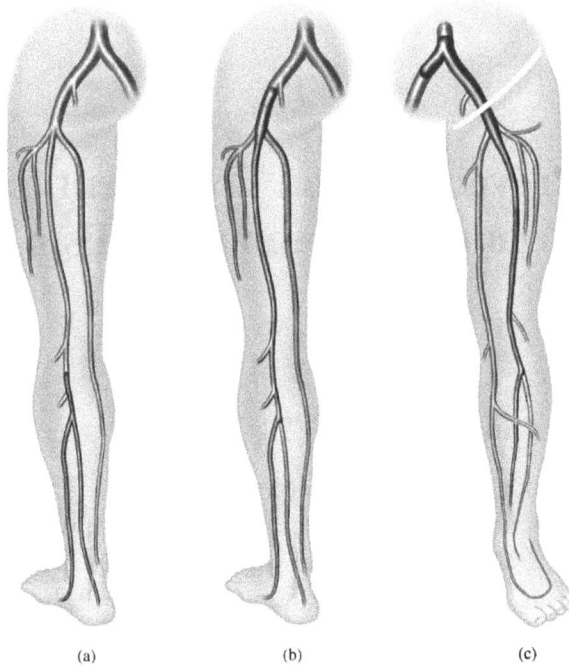

(a)   (b)   (c)

A post-thrombotic syndrome (PTS) may follow important DVTs, particularly thromboses with severe, persisting obstructions at proximal levels (iliacs, femorals, cava). DVT often occurs in the long channels of lower limb veins, in pelvic veins, but it may occur in the veins of the arms (some 10%). However, the risk of embolization from arms is lower as the clot volume that may embolize is small. Arm thrombosis is often associated to compression and tumors and to more complicated clinical cases.

Leg DVT may cause clinically significant PTE more frequently as the clot volume is higher if the femoral veins are affected. Popliteal veins and superficial veins are often affected but, usually, these veins do not produce large volumes of thrombi or emboli; however, a small localized thrombosis may evolve into a full proximal DVT and may propagate to bigger veins increasing the risk for PTE.

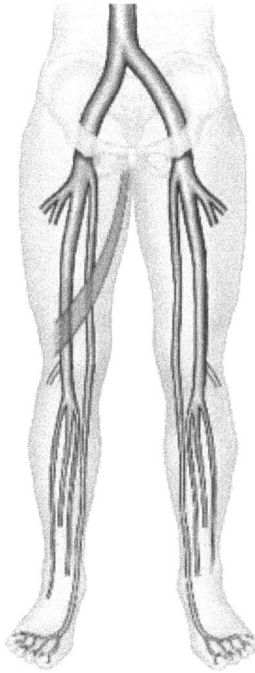

Main deep veins.

Some 50% of patients with DVT may have an occult PTE and some 30% of subjects with PTE have a detectable DVT. Sometimes, the main clot has left the leg for the pulmonary circulation and DVT may be difficult to show in the limbs. In some cases, via a patent foramen ovale (PFO) (Fig. 1), a clot may pass into the arterial circulation and even embolize causing a stroke.

Etiology

Several factors may be involved in the genesis of a thrombus. Oncological conditions may be a concomitant cause particularly in older patients and when thrombosis is recurrent. Screening for tumors is difficult and should be considered on an individual basis. Impaired venous return, immobilization, endothelial injury (after fractures or trauma) coagulation disorders may all be involved in individual combinations.

The Angiology Bible

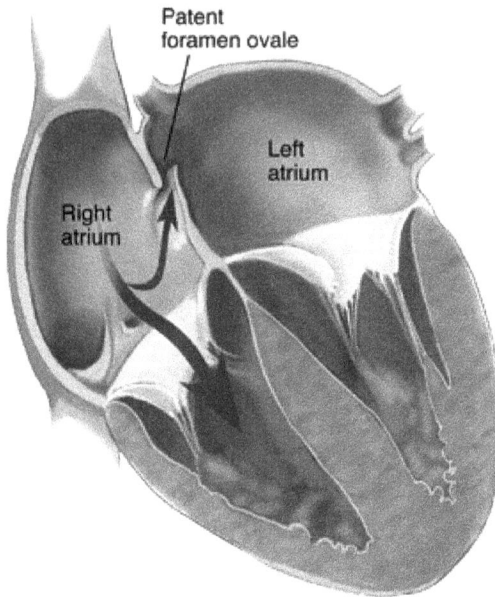

Figure 1. A PFO allows communications between the two atria. Normally, pressure in the right cavity is lower and blood may go from left to right. In case of acute pulmonary hypertension (i.e., for embolism), pressure in the right cavities increases and blood (with clots) may pass into the left cavities. A PFO is common, in possibly 30% of the adult population.

Arm DVT

Catheters, compressions, pacemakers, endovenous injections (including illegal drugs), superior vena cava (SVC) syndrome, subclavian vein compression at the thoracic outlet should be considered as possible causes. Compression by a normal or accessory first rib or fibrous bands (thoracic outlet syndrome), postural conditions in some workers can all contribute to DVT.

Complications

- Obstruction (even phlegmasia, which may lead to venous gangrene)
- Embolization (PTE)

- PTS
- Strokes, TIAs (paradoxical embolism)

These occur when vein emboli pass from the venous into the arterial circulation, generally at cardiac level for a PFO or an abnormal communication. In normal conditions, the pressure in the arterial compartments is higher than in the venous and rarely there is a passage of venous blood into the arterial circulation. In the case of pulmonary embolism, pressure in the pulmonary vessels may be high and venous blood can pass from the right to the left sections of the heart carrying emboli able to cause a stroke.

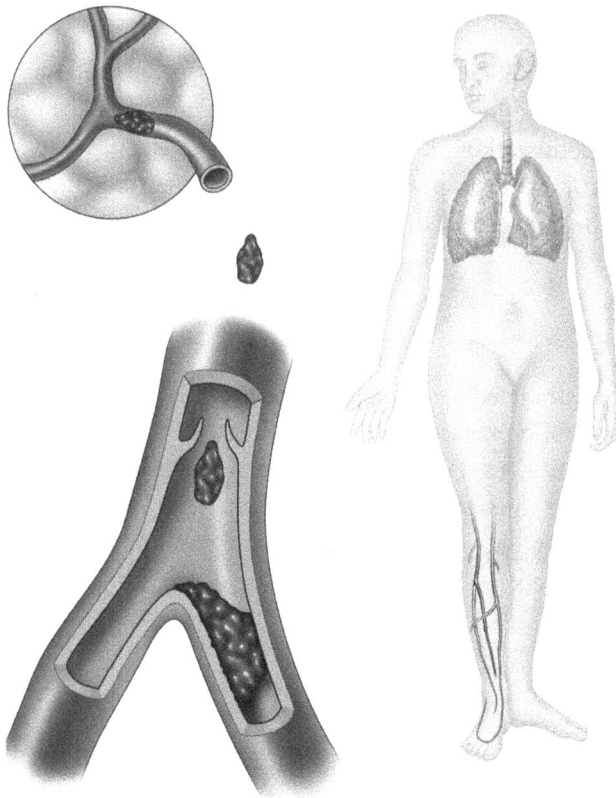

Pulmonary embolism.

Phlegmasia alba may be observed during pregnancy; it is associated to increased venous pressure and tissues swelling that may stop arterial flow and distal perfusion and eventually cause gangrene.

Phlegmasia cerulea (with a bluish skin appearance) is caused by almost total venous occlusion, often caused by compression by a mass (e.g., on the iliac vein). The leg becomes ischemic and cyanotic. Arterial and venous flow stop completely. Gangrene may eventually develop if the condition is left untreated.

Rare infections of thrombosed vein segments (e.g., in the jugular vein, Lemierre Syndrome) may follow tonsillar or pharyngeal infections or periodontal abscesses and neck wounds. Sepsis may follow (with septic embolization). Septic thrombosis after a partum associated to intermittent fever is also possible on rare occasions in less advanced hospitals.

Infective thrombosis may also be caused by catheterization or improper drug injections. Other septic complications may be associated to surgery, immobilization in difficult, complex, hospital patients. While proximal DVT may cause symptoms and asymmetry of the limbs, small distal thrombi can be very difficult to diagnose and detect.

Screening

DVT can be associated to variable symptoms in some patients, spontaneous pain, or pain on bending the leg, tenderness, swelling, redness and a difference in size between limbs with rare observation of fever. All symptoms tend to be more complex in a patient who just had surgery or a trauma. Screening with D-dimer or ultrasound or both is effective in higher-risk subjects.

Chest symptoms

Possible indications of PTE include shortness of breath, chest pain and an unexplained, increased heart rate.

Ultrasound

Scans of the limbs by ultrasound give very reliable information in a matter of minutes and should be considered as soon as possible, particularly in postsurgery patients. The veins are compressed with an ultrasound probe. A patent vein is compressible with limited pressure. A vein including a clot is not easily compressible.

D-dimer is also used as a measurement of some value, particularly after surgery. A low D-dimer value may exclude DVT. Asymmetric swelling due to DVT may also be caused by other causes (compression, cysts, treatments) but none is as dangerous as DVT. Leg pain may be associated with several causes (including local infections). All symptoms require consideration and diagnosis also because some of these lesions (e.g., cellulitis) may be associated to DVT.

A full ultrasound scan is therefore essential and requires only a short interval of time to perform. It is however not a separate test: it is just one part of a full clinical examination. Compressible veins exclude DVT and particularly compressible femoral veins may exclude a proximal DVT which requires urgent attention and anticoagulation.

Compressibility of the femoral veins (with a venous flow clearly phasic with respiration) may exclude major proximal DVT and obstruction in most patients. A clot in the femoral vein (or any big vein) is a dangerous, potential source of large emboli: the observation indicates the need for anticoagulation as soon as possible. Many different types of anticoagulant agents are available to be applied, but in the first instance, priority must be to confirm the presence of a clot.

Popliteal and more distal veins may be more difficult to scan. But the thrombi you cannot easily find with ultrasound are less likely to cause clinically relevant PTEs. Also, iliac veins and cava require a more advanced scanning skill and the evaluation is not always possible. In a situation where the ultrasound scan appears to be negative, it is possible for it to be repeated when a need for further evaluation occurs, as it is completely noninvasive. The test can be made at the bed of the patient and even at home.

Thermography

Thermography is also helpful for screening. Thermal asymmetry and thermic spots raise suspicion on areas that should be immediately scanned with ultrasound. Thermography is fast (images are acquired in seconds), noninvasive and effective but nondiagnostic. An absence of thermal "suspicion areas" may exclude DVT in most patients.

This is also a normal, routine clinical evaluation and not a different, separate test. The separation of clinical evaluation and tests — particularly ultrasound — is not correct, at least not in advanced medicine. It was originally created to produce two different evaluations (with two different costs and revenues). A normal clinical examination now requires the use of ultrasound even at basic levels.

D-dimer derives from the fibrinolysis of clots. Elevated levels tend to indicate the lysis of thrombi. Only the most accurate kits should be used for D-dimer testing. Basically, a negative D-dimer indicates a low probability of DVT and no ultrasonography is needed. However, a positive (high D-dimer) test is not specific. Liver disease, infections, pregnancy, rheumatic disease, inflammation, recent surgery all cause an increase in D-dimer levels.

Clinical problems

The clinical problem is not only to detect the presence of thrombosis: it is essential to define how dangerous the thrombus may be or become. D-dimer may indicate the presence of any thrombus. Ultrasonography indicates the presence of thrombi, their localization and how dangerous the patient's condition is.

In many places, ultrasound scans are much faster than a D-dimer test. In the case of an elevated D-dimer level and a nondiagnostic or clearly negative ultrasound scan, the scan can more easily be repeated. When scans are not possible and the diagnosis is uncertain, we may arbitrarily assume that there is a DVT and treat the patient anyway with anticoagulants, provided there is not a specific risk in using these drugs (e.g., low-molecular-weight heparin (LMWH) is very safe and effective). If further tests are negative, the treatment can be stopped.

Anticoagulation

Anticoagulation (for instance with LMWH or Fondaparinux) — if correctly used — is not dangerous per se. This is not a real treatment but it is a prophylaxis against the extension of the clots and embolization.

Venography as a measurement tool

Venography, at the moment, is practically no longer used, unless some form of invasive treatment is planned. Venography is an invasive procedure in itself, and requires injection of contrast and operator skill, and it may cause side effects.

In rare surgical patients, the evaluation of DVT with venography may be very complex and there are few cases that ultrasound cannot solve. The costs of venography are high and there is a 2% level of complications. Venography is also stressful for patients who may already be under severe clinical stress.

MRI and CT scans also show PTE and possible masses compressing the veins. But venography is still a second level of investigations. In suspected PTE, other tests may be possible (ventilation/perfusion lung scans). However, many tests may delay treatments. It is imperative to start management as soon as possible to avoid the occurrence of embolization. When there are obvious conditions or causes, no other testing is needed after an ultrasound scan and subjects may start immediate anticoagulant treatment.

Hypercoagulability testing in acute phases is controversial; recurrent DVTs, idiopathic thrombosis in subjects without conventional risk factors may indicate the need for testing factors leading to thrombogenicity. When the patient is >40 years and without a history of any thrombotic episode, congenital or genetic factors (even when detected) may have a minimal role in the genesis of a thrombosis. Screening for cancer — associated to unexplained cases of DVT — is difficult and is not considered cost effective. But, it should be considered in individual patients.

Cases 1. Three thermal patterns of DVT. (a) Distal, local and lateral thrombosis. (b) Popliteal thrombosis. (c) Femoral + popliteal thrombosis. The most important observation is asymmetry; thermal images are not diagnostic but guide ultrasound to selected spots.

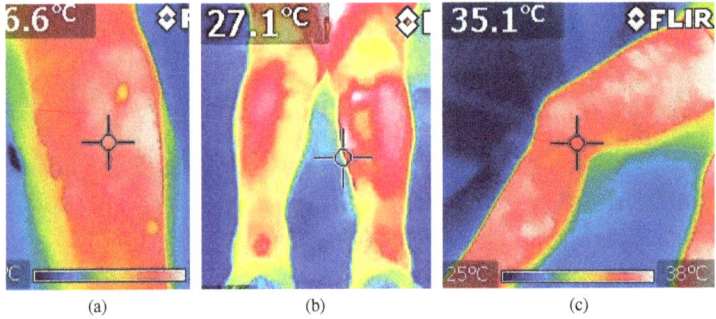

(a)   (b)   (c)

19

DVT Prevention and PTS

DVT prevention

Prevention is based when possible (e.g., in surgical patients) on avoiding immobility or reduced mobility, on mobilizing patients as soon as possible, on controlling the most important risk factors by using LMWH or other anticoagulants. Antithrombotic stockings reduce the volume of stagnant blood in peripheral veins and prevent thrombosis in most lower-risk patients or reduce the risk of thrombotic events. Intermittent pneumatic compression also mobilizes blood in the veins of the lower limbs making DVT less frequent.

Patients should be considered according to their individual risks and to the risks determined by the procedure (minor surgery, average surgical procedure, major surgery). Each procedure defines specific risk conditions: low, medium and high risk for DVT and PTE. The same procedures may have different risks in different types of patients (e.g., very old subjects, diabetics, subjects with neurological deficits, etc.).

The careful, individualized evaluation of patients is a crucial part of DVT prevention, and decisions on method of prevention *should not be made automatically* by placing patients in predefined "risk boxes". For instance, the ability and willingness of the patients to be cooperative or compliant to any particular method of prevention may alter their risk profile.

After surgery, early mobilization, stockings, LMWH used in the period of immobilization reduces the risks of DVT in most patients. LMWH — the most commonly used prevention method — should be tailored on the basis of the patient's weight. Oral anticoagulation (OA) is also used in some patients. OA and aspirin have been used in selected patients but OA increases bleeding risk and aspirin does not seem to be very effective in preventive venous thrombosis.

Antithrombotic stockings and intermittent pneumatic compression can be used in association to anticoagulants or instead of anticoagulation in lower-risk subjects or when anticoagulation is considered dangerous. Intermittent pneumatic compression is not considered to be very effective in some patients (e.g., obese patients).

Stockings in combination with LMWH may be effective for prevention in most low-to-moderate-risk patients and for low-risk procedures. For neurosurgical procedures, the risk of bleeding is very important and specific procedures — not based on anticoagulants — should be considered.

In orthopedics, LMWH, fondaparinux and OA are used as standardized options and should be applied according to individual conditions. Intermittent compression has been effectively used for knee replacement. In these orthopedic patients, the treatment is initially started in advance of surgery and continued for at least 2 weeks or until the patient is completely mobile.

Fondaparinux (once daily) is more effective than LMWH in orthopedic patients and prevents heparin-induced thrombocytopenia (HIT). In cases of very high risk including multiple trauma or multiple surgical procedures, the option of a caval filter before surgery must be considered.

Prevention for medical illness

Several medical conditions causing reduced mobility require DVT prevention. After a stroke, in subjects with metastatic breast cancer (particularly those with central venous catethers), in subjects with mobility problems and handicaps, prophylaxis should be used for individual periods on the basis of the clinical conditions.

Treatment

DVT management, PTE prevention and PTS prevention

For DVT, anticoagulants (heparin) are used at first; then an OA is started within 24–48 h. Most subjects can be treated out of hospital. Elastic compression (better with specific antithrombotic stockings), elevation of the affected limbs, avoiding compression on veins and immobility may all help to improve the condition of the limb.

LMWH is now used in most patients. Unfractionated heparin (UFH) is used only in hospital conditions under careful medical control, as it may cause significant bleeding. LMWH and UFH have basically the same efficacy but LMWHs are much more manageable and expose patients to a lower risk of complications.

Fondaparinux is another subcutaneous heparin that is very effective and does not cause thrombocytopenia. Warfarin and all OA drugs are safe and well known; they are used for different occasions and clinical conditions related to thrombosis. It is important to consider that doses of LMWH should be related to weight. In the case of renal insufficiency, the dosage needs to be adjusted.

As there is no specific relationship between the dose of LMWH and bleeding, no specific monitoring is needed (with routine coagulation tests there are no significant visible changes). Excluding heparin-induced thrombocytopenia (HIT), LMWH may minimally affect the platelet count over time, and it is advisable to check this after 2–3 weeks.

The treatment with heparin is continued until full anticoagulation is reached with OA. However, some patients may only be treated with long-term LMWH (particularly cancer patients). OAs have low costs — excluding the most recent products — and the oral administration make these drugs easy to administer.

Unfractionated heparin may be used instead of LMWH in hospitals. It should be adapted in the case of renal insufficiency (as UFH is not cleared by kidneys). UFH is given in a bolus infusion to reach complete anticoagulation (a partial thromboplastin time (PTT) 1.5–2.5 times the reference range). Treatment is continued until full anticoagulation is reached with OA.

Complications

Bleeding is the most common and important complication of heparin. Thrombocytopenia is rare; UFH may rarely cause skin necrosis. Bleeding due to heparin can be stopped by protamine sulfate. A precise dose should be determined (usually 1 mg of protamine for mg of LMWH in a slow infusion).

Fondaparinux (the selective factor Xa inhibitor) may be used for the initial treatment of DVT or PTE instead of LMWH with comparable modalities. This product is used at fixed doses once daily and does not cause thrombocytopenia; it is therefore used in case of subjects who had an episode of HIT or several administrations of LMWH in previous occasions.

OAs are vitamin K antagonists (these drugs cannot be given to pregnant women); they are used for long-term anticoagulation (3–6 months or more). Doses are lower in older patients and subjects with liver disease. The clinical target is an international normalized ratio (INR) of 2–3, monitored weekly for 3 months. The dose is also adjusted considering drug interactions and bleeding risks and in subjects with transient thrombotic risk conditions, OAs are continued for, usually, 6 months.

The presence of permanent risk factors requires re-evaluation and the continuation of treatment. Repeated DVT episodes also require anticoagulation for longer periods. The risk of bleeding is increased in older patients (70 y+) or with multiple treatments, previous recent MI or strokes, GI bleeding episodes, diabetes. Anemic patients and subjects with renal insufficiency may have an increased risk from bleeding.

The effects of OA can be reversed with vitamin K or by the transfusion of fresh plasma and by prothrombin complex concentrate. In case of overdosage of anticoagulation (INR > 3.4), patients can avoid taking one or more doses or a lower dose according to specific prescriptions.

Warfarin-induced skin necrosis may occur in patients with protein C, S or factor V Leiden mutations. Other anticoagulants can be used, e.g., direct thrombin inhibitors (DTIs, hirudin as lepirudin, bivalirudin, desirudin, argatroban given parenterally; dabigatran per os). Oral factor Xa inhibitors (e.g., rivaroxaban and apixaban) are now usable for the management of anticoagulation in DVT.

In summary, one LMWH and one OA may treat most patients (96%). Each center should define its policy in the use of these products. Using the same products for most patients allows a building up of specific experience and confidence in the products.

Lysis

Streptokinase, urokinase and alteplase lyse clots reducing the impact of PTS. The risks of bleeding are high. The main indication for lysis is the presence of large proximal thrombi at the iliofemoral veins causing severe obstructions and a high risk for phlegmasia. A local perfusion with catheter is generally better than a systemic IV infusion. Lysis is problematic in surgical patients or subjects with recent bleeding.

Caval filters (IVC filters or IVCFs) prevent PTE when:

(a) anticoagulants are not possible or ineffective
(b) embolization continues even under full anticoagulation.

When placed below the level of the renal veins by catheterization, the caval filter blocks possible pulmonary emboli. Some filters are removable and can be used on a temporary basis. Filters may have long-term complications (dislocation, obstruction of the lower vena cava and even venous gangrene, renal failure) but it must be considered that this measure is used in difficult conditions, in difficult patients with justified risks. Dislodged IVCFs need surgery or removal by catheter.

Surgical removal of thrombi

Surgery for thrombus removal is now used only in rare cases. Thrombectomy, fasciotomy may be used for cases with impending or clear phlegmasia, not responding to other medical treatment and in subjects with high risk of venous gangrene.

Post-thrombotic syndrome (PTS)

The prevention of the PTS — a more serious and progressively aggravating form of CVI — after a significant DVT episode (e.g., femoral thrombosis) includes mobilization, exercise, periodic leg elevation and stockings with some 30–40 mmHg of compression.

Obstruction and high venous pressure after a DVT cause important damages to the deep venous system. Valvular cusps involved in the thrombosed segments are badly damaged or destroyed in the process leading to thrombus lysis and in the following revascularization phase. The occurrence of rethrombosis in the segment may produce further severe damage.

Guidelines

There are documents to use as guidelines for thrombosis management and prevention. The following document includes detailed instructions for single applications of DVT/PTE prophylaxis and management.

> Nicolaides AN, Fareed J, Kakkar AK, Comerota AJ, Goldhaber SZ, Hull R *et al.* Prevention and treatment of venous thromboembolism — International Consensus Statement. *Int. Angiol.*, 2013, 32(2): 111–260.

Comment

There is an approach that tends to "industrialize" medicine, standardizing patients with the main excuse of controlling costs. In this field (DVT/PTE prevention), it is possible to standardize but not all elements. The individual value of each single patient and clinical case should be always considered with attention by physicians.

Prevention and therapy for every patient should be decided by doctors and not by managers or simply by protocols. Prescription is always an individual action and a precise right and service. The prevention of DVT/PTE and the field of anticoagulants is a huge, expanding business. We must be very careful to avoid an "industrial" view and standardization abuses and we cannot miss individual needs.

Case 1. Compression of the right iliac artery onto the left iliac vein may be a cause of recurrent thrombosis, particularly in women, to be considered when thrombosis recurs on the left side. The compression (with the section of the vein indicated) may range from (a) a partial one which does not affect flow to (d) total occlusion.

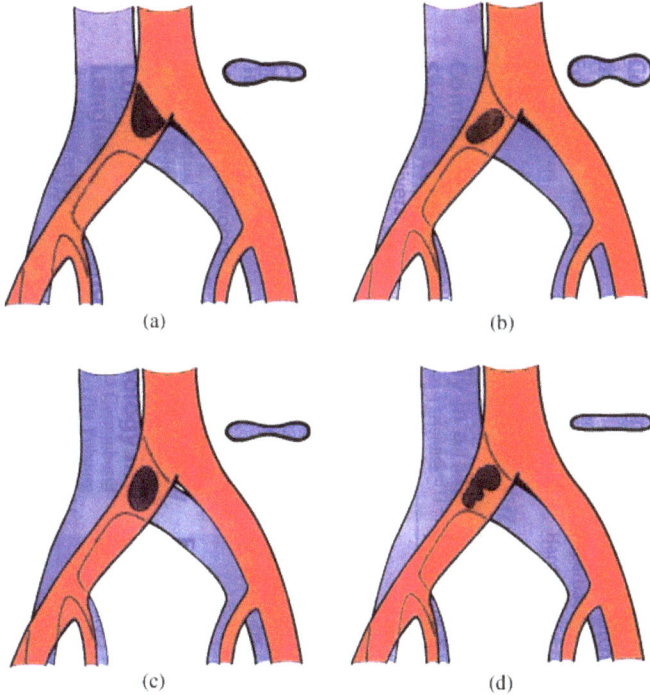

(a)

(b)

(c)

(d)

20

Chronic Venous Insufficiency

Introduction

Chronic venous insufficiency (CVI) can be caused by congenital venous and valvular abnormalities, PTS, untreated or complicated VV and by AV communications (in a limited number of cases).

Chronic increase in venous pressure is eventually transferred from the larger veins to capillary levels, creating a condition of venous hypertensive microangiopathy characterized by a massive dilatation of capillaries that become glomerular-like: this transformation greatly increases their exchange surface with excessive filtration of fluids and protein into the interstitial space filled with "gel matrix" that greatly changes its composition (Fig. 1). The proteins and protein degradation product tend to stay in the interstitial fluid and increase local osmolarity which attracts more water from the microcirculation.

Distal lymphatic capillaries and very small veins are compressed or obstructed in the extracapillary space and do not drain the extra fluids, increasing the edema in the area. Slow flow decreases the rate of delivery of oxygen; CO_2 increases as it is not cleared from the interstitial space. High levels of CO_2 tend to cause an increase in local vasodilatation.

Edema separates cells from their nutritional sources (the capillaries) and the nutrition of tissues becomes critical. Eventually relative to ischemia and edema, nutritional alterations create a deadly combination.

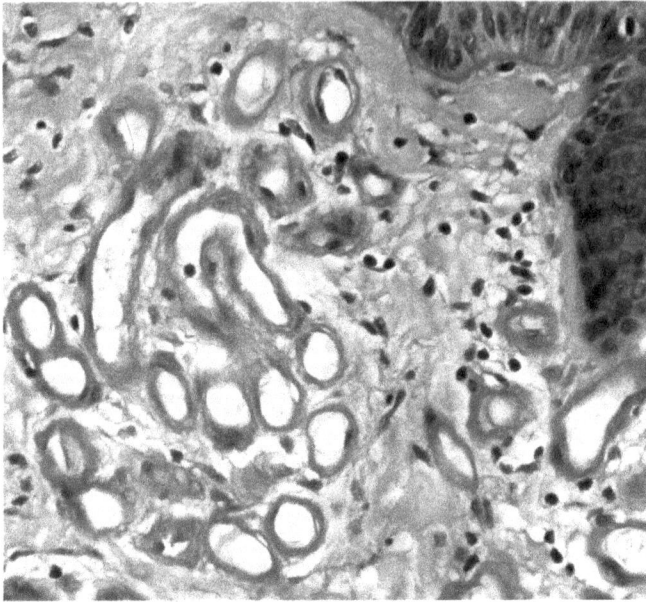

Figure 1.   Dilatation of capillaries in a glomerular-like aspect in the skin of a patient with CVI and initial ulceration. The large capillary network allows great filtration of fluids into the extracapillary space with formation of edema.

Any small trauma may cause a significant damage to the tissues and the skin and eventually evolve into skin breaks and ulcerations, which can prove very difficult to heal.

Exercise — e.g., walking, running, swimming — lowers distal venous pressure. Muscular pump dysfunction and valvular incompetence or absence (associated to chronic reflux) tend to increase pressure producing a condition of chronic venous hypertension. CVI when multiplied by years of high capillary pressure causes progressive skin changes.

Some 30% of patients, during the 5–10 years after a thrombosis develop PTS. But it depends on the care used for the thrombotic event and the postthrombotic management. The social environment, education, access to healthcare, income, and even neglect are part of the equation. In some cases, a postthrombotic condition is visible in less than

12 months. Deep venous incompetence may be associated to selective incompetence of some perforating veins in more than 30% of the patients.

Any outflow obstruction increases venous pressure. During exercise, outflow — if blocked — may cause venous engorgement with dilatation of the distal system and muscular pain (decreasing with rest) constituting venous claudication.

The progressive CVI skin changes in the perimalleolar regions, particularly the internal regions, stain the skin with hemosiderin and blood degradation products. The accumulation of proteins makes the skin thicker, less flexible and more prone to the effects of any minimal trauma. Hemosiderin and its debris are considered the main cause of the brownish colorations that the skin may assume.

Venous hypertensive microangiopathy

The glomerular-like evolution (Fig. 1) of the distal capillaries with edema and reduced nutritional perfusion are progressive. In time, edema becomes fibrosis, with significant loss of perfusion of the nutritional layers while the global and thermoregulatory layers show (for instance by laser Doppler flowmetry) a paradoxical global increase in flow and perfusion.

Minimal trauma, small cuts leading to ulcerations, edema, discoloration, ulcerations, pain (often minimal when the skin is intact), the association with primary or secondary varicose veins are all part of a complex individual clinical picture.

Ultrasound scans show obstruction and incompetence levels and detect the incompetent, superficial venous sites that can be treated. The function of some venous valves should be evaluated with attention as some can be restored. Obstruction can be quantified by plethysmography and severe outflow problems may need venography — if surgery is considered.

Ambulatory venous pressure (AVP) measurements are the basis of all venous physiology. A small needle in a distal vein and a pressure recorder show the variations of the pressure curve and the refilling time (RT = the time needed to the venous system to refill from the arterial,

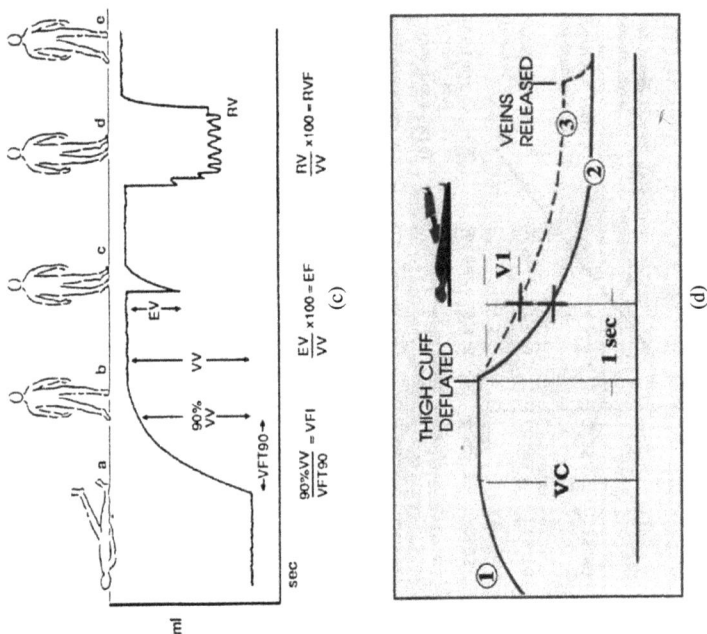

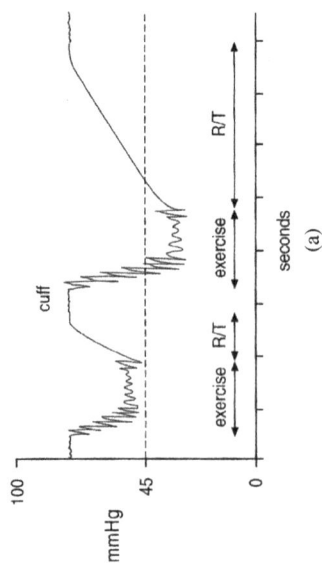

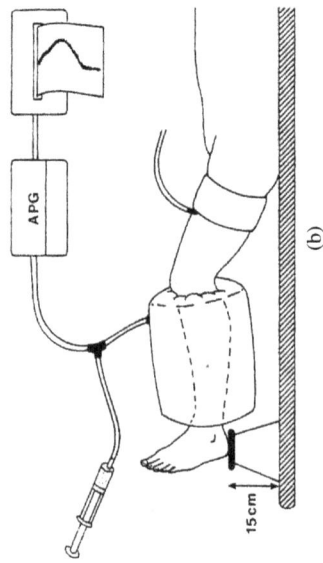

Figure 2. APG is used to quantitatively assess limbs in CVI. (a) AVP measurements with and without a cuff excluding the superficial system. (b) The air plethysmograph. The 100 mL syringe included in the circuit is used for volume calibration. (c) The maneuvers and methods of deriving the APG measurements. Both the superficial system and the deep system can be evaluated. (d) The venous flow curve indicating the presence of deep venous obstruction. (1) Inflow curve, (2) outflow (normal) and (3) outflow decreased by obstruction. VC = venous capacitance.

distal side). A fast refilling time is associated to filling from the proximal venous segments with reflux. The method is useful to classify patients for venous studies.

Venous pressure values (AVP) and RT are the basis for the evaluation of any form of management. Pressure should normalize and RT should become longer (>16–18 mmHg) to have a real improvement in venous hypertension and CVI.

Air plethysmography (APG) (Figs. 2(a)–2(c)) can also be used for a full noninvasive evaluation of the dynamics of the venous system — comparable to AVP measurements — including the measurement of the obstruction entity and level.

Invasive methods

Descending venography is invasive and complex, but it is still used to study valves when an intervention is planned. Its use is limited to selected patients likely to be treated with reconstructive venous surgery.

Vein management in CVI: A summary

Wherever possible in CVI, subjects should be treated with the aim of preventing an evolution to more severe levels of venous hypertension. Treatment should consider the following points:

- It is important to treat all significant incompetent points (those that change AVP or RT) with surgery or sclerotherapy.
- The management is always based on compression and exercise.
- All ulcerations improve reducing venous pressure with compression, treating local infections and with the correct medications.
- Surgery may be limited and repeated in time, in small interventions, in well-selected patients and it should be alternate to sclerotherapy if needed.
- The treatment of all incompetent superficial venous communications with surgery or sclerotherapy corrects most of the incompetence even in predominantly deep venous incompetence.

- The transplant of the incompetent segments with competent veins may be effective for a long time (some vein transplants are effective even after 40 years).
- External valvuloplasty — with present and functional cusps — is a very good option.
- It is important to avoid excesses in complicating surgery or sclerotherapy.
- The key for patients with a chronic disease such as CVI is a chronic treatment (e.g., dentist's technique) consisting of repeated, minimal, invasive procedures.
- Iliac compression is not so common and stenting — now fashionable — may be reserved to some specific subjects with severe obstruction.
- In some positions, the iliac veins always appear compressed.
- Most venous ulcers are associated to lack of attention and are a sign of neglect. Continuous care and attention are needed to heal most ulcers.

21

Superficial Venous Thrombosis

Introduction

Superficial venous thrombosis (SVT) may occur spontaneously in subjects with a subclinical, hidden condition (e.g., diseases like Behçet's or in oncological conditions) (see Fig. 1). Intravenous therapy can produce a thrombosis or an inflammatory reaction without thrombosis (phlebitis) or thrombosis and inflammation or infection may be concomitant (thrombophlebitis). SVT occurring in different places without previous venous disease suggests the presence of some hidden, systemic problems (e.g., pancreatic carcinoma).

In VV, a small trauma or a compression may produce thrombosis in a dilated, enlarged superficial vein. The saphenous vein and its branches — the larger superficial veins — are most frequently affected. A concomitant DVT may be present in some 30% of patients with lower limb SVT.

Localized pain, an incompressible vein which looks and feels like a cord are common observations. Often the thrombosed vein can appear prominent and upon elevation of the leg, this prominence is still visible/present. In some cases, often associated with infection, systemic signs (fever, elevated white cell count) may also be present.

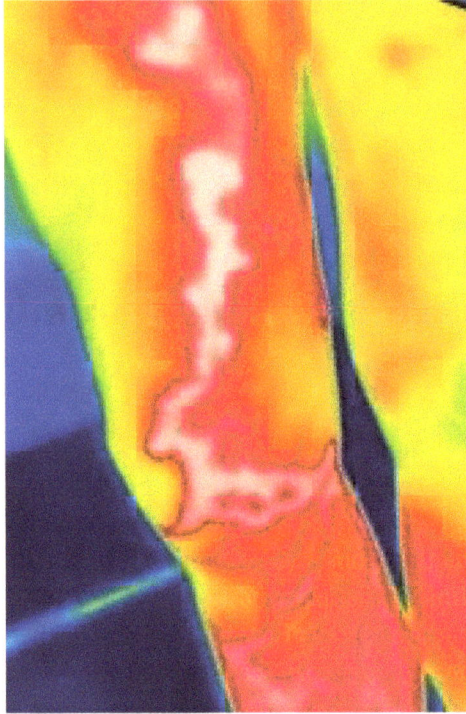

Figure 1.   Superficial venous thrombosis.

Differential diagnoses

Erythema nodosum occasionally may give a similar appearance; also, cellulitis, lymphangitis or traumas, rupture of a Baker's cyst (distally to the knee) may mimic SVT but, usually, the diagnosis is clear (Fig. 1).

Thermal and ultrasonic evaluation

Thermography clearly shows the extension, localization and patterns of the inflamed veins. Ultrasound scans may evaluate in seconds the deep and venous system and the possible extension into the deep venous system (e.g., at the SFJ).

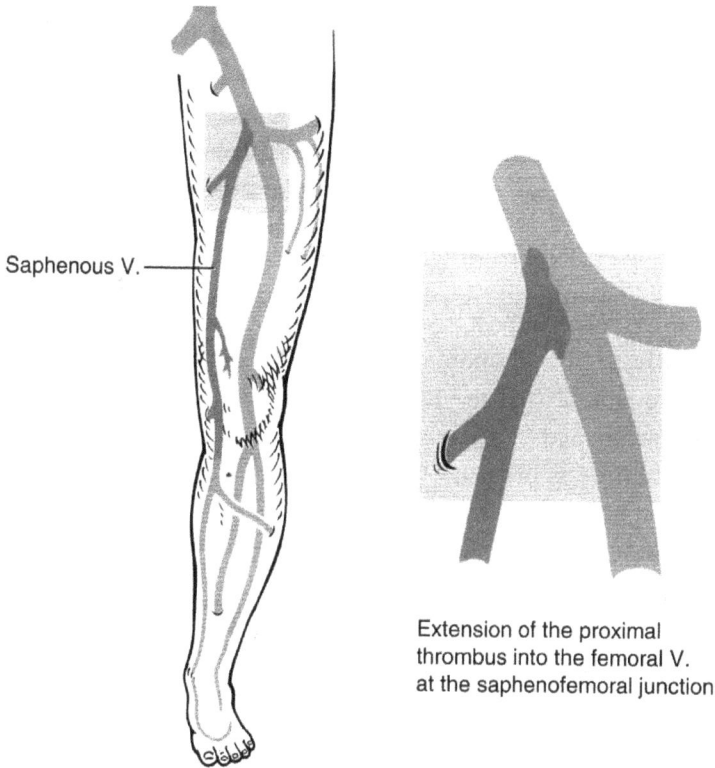

Extension of the proximal
thrombus into the femoral V.
at the saphenofemoral junction

Figure 2.   Extension of a thrombus from the superficial to the deep venous system.

Management of SVT

Local or systemic treatment for pain, compression, heat limb mobilization is the key aspect of management. The thrombus can be squeezed out with small cuts on the vein if needed under local anesthetic.

Progressive extension of a thrombus in the long saphenous vein into the deep system may indicate the need for surgical ligation of the greater saphenous vein to stop progress of the thrombus into the deep system (Fig. 2).

LMWHs improve symptoms and make resolution of SVT faster. LMWH is also a prophylaxis against progression into deep veins and the evolution or a concomitant development of DVT.

For SVT, individual management is the basis of a most successful outcome for the patient. Excision of the vein with the thrombus (with other varicosities) can be done, but it is better to wait for the resolution of the symptoms before surgery. Usually, compression and pain management are very effective.

The thrombosed vein can also be punctured (under local anesthetic) with a fine blade and the thrombus, if recent, can be easily squeezed out. Elimination of the thrombus or a significant amount of it tends to cause the pain to decrease and helps with a much faster healing process. A clinically significant postthrombotic episode after an SVT is considered rare unless there is an associated DVT. Management of SVT must also consider risk factors and hypercoagulability.

Fondaparinux is particularly effective in SVT making the resolution faster and in preventing immediate recurrences or extensions. For long segments of the greater saphenous veins, excision/stripping of the segment may be needed to control symptoms. Ligation of the SFJ blocks the extension into the deep system and LMWHs and compression minimize complications.

A short word about septic thrombophlebitis

Septic thrombophlebitis is now rare in advanced healthcare systems. Where it occurs, antibiotic treatment and removal of septic segments (if possible) are the best solutions. Any catheter, when there is a phlebitis or SVT, should be removed. Conservative management and medical treatment help to solve the problem. Thrombectomy with catheters, in selected cases, is possible according to anatomical localization.

22

Axillary and Subclavian Thrombosis (Arm DVT)

Introduction

This type of thrombosis is not very common (some 10% or less of these patients may have a PTE). After a thrombosis of the veins of the arm/shoulder, recurrent DVT is common if there is an anatomical cause. In the Paget–Schroetter syndrome, arm thrombosis is associated to efforts and extreme positions of the arm.

Thrombosis may also be associated to neurological symptoms. The subclavian vein may be compressed between a first rib, the anterior scalene muscle posteriorly and the clavicle. Costoclavicular ligaments may get inserted more laterally causing compression of the subclavian vein.

However, the occurrence of arm DVT in some patients may be associated to thrombophilia. Secondary thrombosis is associated to catheters, nonvascular compressions, pacemakers, endovenous injections (including illegal drugs), SVC syndrome; subclavian vein compression at the thoracic outlet should be considered as a possible cause.

The compression by a normal or accessory first rib or by fibrous bands (thoracic outlet syndrome), repetitive, postural working conditions can all contribute to arm DVT. For young athletes, repetitive extreme amounts of exercise may lead to hyperabduction; and irregular healing after fractures or surgery and may cause DVT.

Symptoms of axillary thrombosis

Symptoms are usually clear with edema, swelling, pain, cyanosis and the appearance of collateral veins at the shoulder in some patients. Neurological symptoms (involving nerve compression at C8-T1) and onto the brachial plexus may cause several problems including muscle loss, pain, altered motion and sensitivity at the arm and hands.

Diagnostic techniques

The diagnosis, usually clinical, is confirmed by duplex scanning to show occlusion. However, detecting the obstruction is just the first step. MRI may help define anatomy of the region and possible compression or bending of the veins. MRI may be repeated in different positions to show the effects of compression with the motion of the arm (Fig. 1). Chest X-ray (or CT scans) must exclude cervical ribs, possible compression from tumors or lymph nodes and more complex intrathoracic problems.

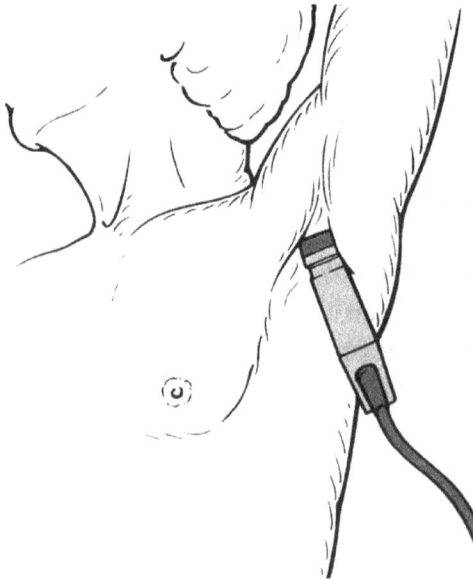

Figure 1.   Evaluation of an axillary thrombosis.

Management

Primary treatment with thrombus-catheter-directed thrombolysis is very effective, if possible, within 2 weeks from the thrombus formation. This procedure at the arm has a relatively low risk of bleeding. Most patients have a good outcome with conservative medical treatment including anticoagulants.

Surgical correction of compressions includes anterior scalenectomy, the resection of the first rib and debridement of the vein from inflamed, compressive, surrounding tissues. The transaxillary approach minimizes neurological risks but rib resections may be more difficult or incomplete. In acute occlusions, the resection of the anterior scalene and the first rib with venolysis is better than thrombectomy or thrombolysis with catheters.

Bypass of the obstructed venous segment with the LSV has been attempted with good results in selected patients. The most frequent approach is a conservative management with anticoagulants and exercise. Surgery is used in more complex or repetitive cases, younger subjects and when there are no concomitant oncological conditions.

The duration of the anticoagulant treatment is not clear. When there is no compression and the vein appears free from external conditioning, the thrombophilic state may be considered. But the therapy is always anticoagulants.

In the matter of secondary thrombosis, it is important to remove all catheters. Repeated thrombosis with no clear explanation requires screening for hidden systemic or oncological conditions. The survival of subjects with arm/axillary thrombosis is lower than the survival for comparable subjects with lower limbs DVT as this condition may be an expression of a subclinical condition.

23

Pulmonary Thromboembolism

Introduction

With some 50,000 confirmed deaths a year in the USA, pulmonary thromboembolism (PTE) is one of the most important preventable clinical conditions. It is possible that many more cases of unexplained sudden death may be caused by PTE. It is currently considered the third leading cause of death in hospitalized patients. A confirmed diagnosis of DVT is evident in some 30% of patients with PTE and it is clear that preventing DVT also prevents PTE. Pulmonary emboli also derive from venous catheters and often follow any type of surgery and particularly operations involving large veins.

Embolization from amniotic fluid may occur during labor. Also "fat" emboli from fractured long bones may cause PTE with respiratory insufficiency, petechial rash (upper body), coagulopathy and even encephalopathy (with a PFO, even strokes are possible). Less common now are septic emboli, embolization from an atrial myxoma, the extension into the IVC of a renal cell carcinoma. Some 60% of untreated proximal DVTs may produce a clinical significant PTE while <10% of PTE may produce pulmonary infarctions.

Symptoms

Nonspecific symptoms are observed particularly in subjects with cardiovascular disease. Dyspnea, chest pain, hemoptysis are present in only 15%

of patients with PTE. Dyspnea and chest pain can even be absent in some 25% of patients with PTE.

Tachycardia, tachypnea, an altered mental status are all symptoms suggestive of PTE in high-risk subjects. Pleural friction and a pleural effusion (on X-ray) and a S1Q3T3 EKG morphology are not very common (<10%) and often limited.

Diagnostic and imaging

A chest X-ray may appear normal at the beginning, or it may show a pleural cap. Atrial fibrillation, nonspecific ST and T wave, acute and unexplained sinus tachycardia, right heart strain coronary ischemia may all be present and should be put into context. Arterial blood gas evaluation reveals hypoxia, respiratory alkalosis, increased arterial–alveolar oxygen gradient. The D-dimer can be increased when DVT is present but it is specific for PTE.

Troponins may be elevated in acute, massive–submassive PE causing hemodynamic instability (with systolic blood pressure <90 mmHg), right heart strain leading to myocardial ischemia. Plasma B-type natriuretic peptide may be elevated in right heart strain (but it is nonspecific for this condition). CTA is the preferred option (if available) and the patient can be scanned in a short time.

More accurate are ventilation-perfusion scans and angiography if the patient is stable enough to undergo the test. When contrast agents are not advisable, an echocardiogram shows the right heart dysfunction as a significant indication of PE. Intravascular ultrasound (IVUS) is also used as a more advanced method if there is time, if the patient is stable and if there is a possibility of sucking out or lysing the thrombus.

Treatment

Rapid anticoagulation is the best option but this is of course always dependent upon clinical conditions. Heparin, LMWH or Fondaparinux as soon as possible after stabilization therapy is effective. Thrombolysis, when and if possible, is considered effective for large clots in subjects with right heart failure. The clinical picture tends to improve in 24 h. The cost of lysis and the risk of bleeding are generally high.

IVC interruption with filters must be considered when embolization continues despite adequate anticoagulant management or when anticoagulants are not possible. Caval filters can be used prophylactically in very high-risk, not otherwise treatable patients. IVC filters are always used with anticoagulation particularly in cancer patients.

Temporary filters are available. Filters can now be placed using ultrasound or IVUS via the common femoral vein or the jugular vein. Angiography of the cava is generally needed to show caval thrombi, possible duplications and the position of the renal veins and collaterals. Recurrence of DVT may be more common in patients with filters.

Surgical treatment

Consideration of surgical treatment may be given in the case of patients who are very unstable, after failing medical therapy, but have good prospects of survival — particularly subjects with persisting, severe hypotension or those after a failed catheter-directed lysis attempt. Subjects with tumors and/or foreign body emboli may also be considered for treatment with open surgery. Suction embolectomy devices are reducing the need for surgery.

Prognosis

PTE is the cause of preventable hospital deaths many of which can be avoided by proper initial management of DVT risks and by the screening of higher-risk patients. Decreasing risk of embolism is the key element to effective management of DVT and PTE. IVC filters are useful for secondary prevention of embolization but do not affect thrombosis.

Multiple episodes of embolization eventually produce a chronic pulmonary disease. Finding emboli in lung vessels (e.g., with CT scans) in patients with no symptoms or with minimal symptoms does not constitute PE but it is a "normal" evolution of most thrombi that eventually break into small parts and are lysed in the lung circulation.

24

Vascular Andrology, PCS, Vulvar Varices

Vascular erectile dysfunction

Erectile dysfunction (ED) may be related to several factors, some of vascular origin, almost all with a vascular component. It is generally common in aging men and it is basically related to a natural decrease in the production of testosterone. ED may be concomitant or may be aggravated by the classic vascular risk factors (particularly smoking). Several treatments are now available. Modern management of ED is very effective.

ED is caused by a combination of vascular and neurological disorders, could be a complication of surgery, diabetes and diabetic microangiopathy and is generally associated to hormonal problems (the most frequent is a decrease in testosterone). In the recent past, the most common cause of ED was considered to be diffuse atherosclerosis and a block of the penile arteries. Several bypass procedures were attempted.

Actually, most patients with ED have a limited organic vascular component as the arteries appear normal. However, the mechanism linked to vasodilatation, engorgement and erection appear to be altered particularly from a functional point of view. Atherosclerosis and aging may decrease the capacity of vasodilatation.

The endothelial function, microvascular reactivity and smooth muscle relaxation are altered when the level of testosterone decreases. Functional alterations may limit the amount of blood captured by the premicrocirculation arteries, and in some cases, venous outflow may also be altered causing a fast leak of blood from the engorged compartment with a failure to maintain tumescence.

In subjects with sickle cell anemia, spinal cord injuries or hypogonadism, this mechanism is altered. Several drugs may cause ED but ED may often happen without a real or significant vascular component. Alcohol may temporarily alter ED.

Clinical evaluation

The evaluation of the traditional risk factors and hormonal patterns (testosterone being the most important) are associated to a full evaluation excluding screening for depression. This may be the first real sign of aging for most men and it is an occasion to check all risk conditions.

Very often, men are more preoccupied for a minor level of ED than for angina. Anatomical penile abnormalities and plaques causing fibrosis should therefore be evaluated and seen with ultrasound. The presence of diffuse atherosclerosis (carotid, aorta, femoral arteries) should be seen in the same session and may offer a different perspective.

Organic ED is associated to absence of nocturnal erections or erections on awakening which may be present in patients with psychological problems (these are generally younger). Hormonal assessment is essential. If testosterone levels are low, a correction may be needed. But ED is not treated by simply restoring the levels of testosterone. Thyroid function, possible diabetes and atheromas need full evaluation.

A penile–brachial pressure comparison is not very useful and a real obstruction at the penile arteries tends to be a late occurrence in older subjects or in patients with very bad risk condition levels. Duplex ultrasound shows penile morphology and flow characteristics.

Treatment

The treatment of ED, including the management of all risk conditions, is based on specific drug treatment. Oral phosphodiesterase (PDE) inhibitors and oral apomorphine, intracavernous injections of PGE1 (or intramural application of the same prostaglandins) tend to be effective in most patients. Oral PDE inhibitors inhibit guanosine monophosphate (cGMP), the specific PDE (PDE5), the predominant PDE isoform in the penile circulation.

Sildenafil, vardenafil, tadalafil increase cGMP and appear to enhance the nitric oxide release essential for erection. The side effects are comparable for all these drugs and all three are almost equally effective when used at least 1 h before the intercourse. All these drugs cause coronary dilatation and may potentiate the hypotensive effects of other nitrates. Therefore, nitrates are a contraindication for 24 h after the administration of ED drugs. Collateral effects also include visual (retinal perfusion) abnormalities, headache, flushing and tachycardia.

Tadalafil has been linked to myalgias. Some PDE5 users have developed anterior ischemic optic neuropathy and retinal perfusional problems. Vardenafil must be used with attention in subjects using alfa-blockers as they may cause prolonged hypotension. Sildenafil when administered with doxazosin appears to be safe. Apomorphine improves nervous conduction and signals from and to the central nervous system. It is moderately effective although it may cause nausea and hypotension. Alprostadil (PGE1) is used for intraureteral administration or for intra-cavernosal injections. PGE1 may cause priapism in some patients and some pain.

Surgical options for erectile dysfunction

Surgical options in subjects not responding to therapy now include prostheses; revascularization procedures have been used less frequently in the last few years.

Conclusion

In conclusion, erectile dysfunction cannot be considered simply a vascular problem (it is more a functional vascular–nervous–microcirculatory disease) and definitely it is not associated in most patients with a vascular occlusive disorder.

ED is the ultimate and possibly the best demonstration of endothelial dysfunction, very often the only one that can be documented, as the penile circulation is the most sensitive circulation to be affected — and in an early phase — by endothelial function alterations.

Varicocele

Diagnosis

- Enlarged veins in the spermatic cord (usually left)
- Pain, tension at the left hemiscrotum
- Reflux in the spermatic veins
- Infertility in some patients

Introduction

Varicocele (Fig. 1) is characterized by varicosities of the pampiniform plexus. It is due to incompetence or absence of valves in the spermatic and testicular vein (see Case 1(a)). The hydrostatic venous pressure is transmitted to the spermatic cord causing distension and tortuosity of the pampiniform plexus. Most often (90%), varicocele is present on the left side where the termination of the spermatic vein into the left renal vein allows more direct transmission of retrograde pressure along the incompetent vein to the scrotum. In the case of a gross varicocele, the spermatic cord is distended by multiple veins which are visible and palpable. The definition of varicocele implies that there is venous incompetence allowing reflux of blood from the great veins into the plexus.

It is possible to have dilated veins without incompetence and vice versa. Clinically overt varicocele is easy to diagnose and evaluate and enlarged veins may be palpated with the patient standing and are often said to feel like a "bag of worms". If the patient is only examined lying down, then the diagnosis may be missed. The testis appears enlarged and patients may complain of a dragging scrotal sensation. Mild, asymptomatic varicocele may be unassociated with signs/symptoms and difficult to detect clinically. Varicocele in its clinical and subclinical forms is considered to be a possible, important cause of male infertility, especially if bilateral. Sudden onset of varicocele in older patients may be caused by

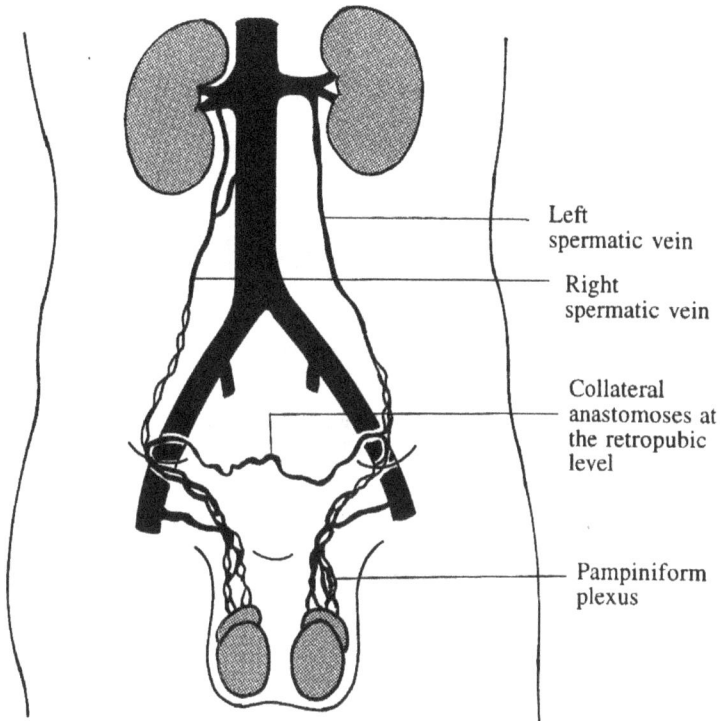

Figure 1. Varicocele.

an obstruction of the left renal vein by a carcinoma of the kidney. If suspected, an ultrasound scan will usually confirm the diagnosis.

The diagnosis of varicocele is now usually made with B-mode ultrasound scanning which indicates the presence of dilated veins, increasing in size during a Valsalva maneuver or by standing. Color duplex scanning visualizes the veins and demonstrates retrograde reflux. Reflux in the spermatic plexus is first evaluated and shown with the patient supine, fully relaxed, performing a Valsalva maneuver (see Case 1(b)).

The reflux in the spermatic plexus is visible during Valsalva. Reflux is often transmitted distally to the veins surrounding the testis. In case of a lack of demonstrable reflux in the supine position, the test may be repeated with the patient standing. The hemodynamic problem is clinically relevant when associated with low sperm count.

Case 1. Thermographic cases of varicocele.

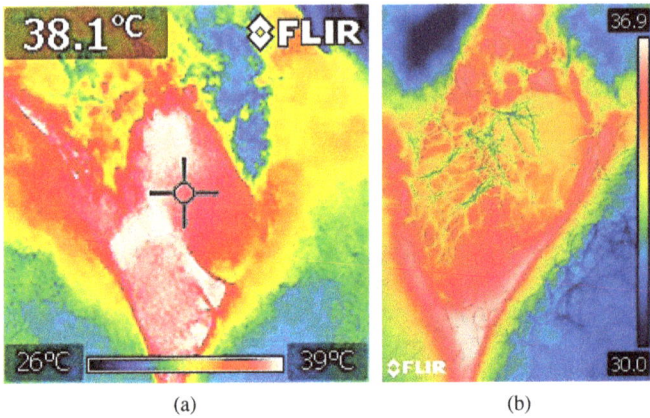

(a)   (b)

Pelvic congestion syndrome and vulvar varices

Diagnosis

- Pelvic pain
- Vulvar varicosities
- Ovarian vein reflux

Introduction

The pelvic congestion syndrome (PCS) (Fig. 2) is often unrecognized or poorly treated, and patients are treated by different specialists for the two main problems present: pelvic pain and vulvar varicosities. Vulvar vari-cose veins (VV) are a relatively common disorder, sometimes associated with pelvic pain, but they are not necessarily related to PCS. The anatomy of the ovarian veins is shown in Fig. 2. Vulvar varicosity may be associ-ated with the features outlined as A–D in this figure.

The etiology of vulvar VV has been considered to be an equivalent to PTS in the legs. Following pregnancy, some of the divisions of the internal iliac veins may occlude and the resulting outflow obstruction produces signs and symptoms similar to the PTS in the leg. Perivulvular varices are com-mon during pregnancy, but they usually disappear after delivery. The sudden appearance of vulvar VV during the third or fourth month of the second or third pregnancy may indicate a pelvic vein thrombosis.

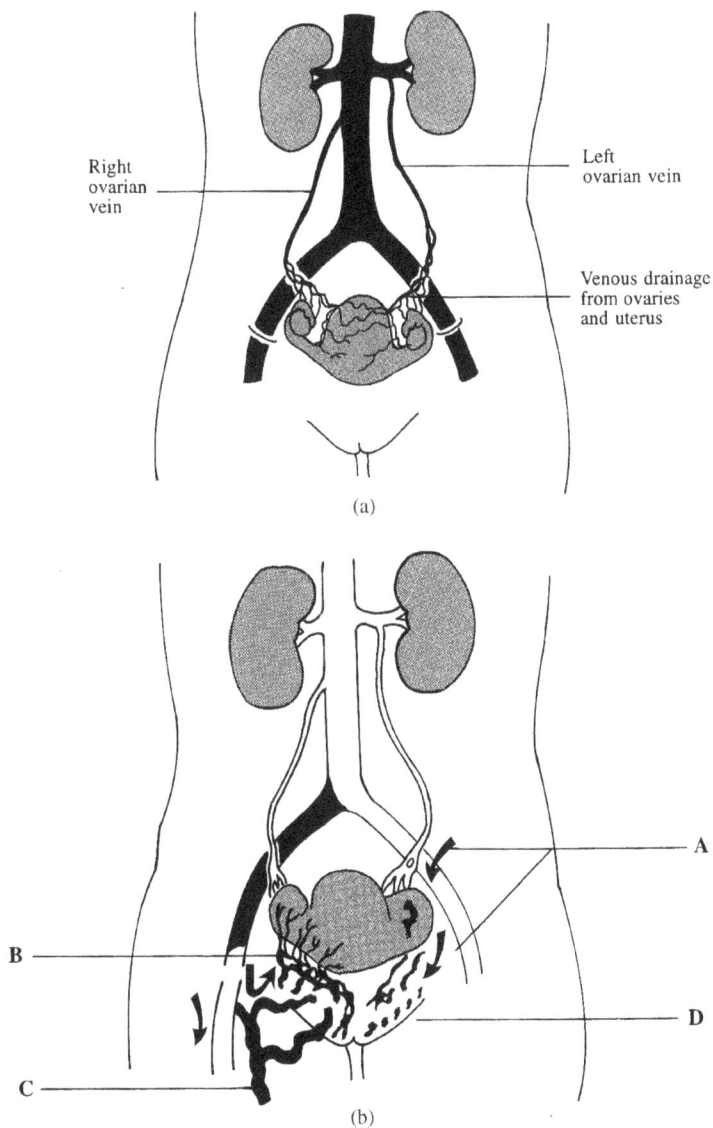

Figure 2. The pelvic congestion syndrome. (a) Intra-abdominal PCS (mainly congenital). (b) PCS with connections to the superficial venous system (possibly postthrombotic). Types of connection: (1) to the iliac veins, (2) to the ovarian veins, (3) to the LSV and (4) intralabial veins. A — True varicocele (reflux in the ovarian vein, particularly the left one. B — Secondary venous distension due to iliac or pelvic obstruction. C — Severe reflux and venous hypertension at the level of the femoral vein, LSV and its medial collaterals. D — Localized varicosities associated with cavernosal tissue and sometimes with little AV communications.

In some patients, vulvar varices persist and increase in size with subsequent pregnancies. They may extend to the posterior part of the leg and thigh. It is possible that PCS is associated with consequences of a DVT, but it is also possible that simple, pure ovarian vein reflux may be the basis of the disorder.

PCS is characterized by pain of variable intensity which is worse premenstrually, and it is increased by fatigue, standing, and during or after intercourse. These symptoms are often associated with vulvar varicosities. Also "broad ligament varicocele" has been associated with chronic pelvic pain in multiparous women. Pelvic varicosities exist when the ovarian veins are congenitally incompetent, causing a situation which is analogous to scrotal varicocele in men.

Diagnosis

On examination of patients with PCS, atypical veins are seen to be present on the back of the thigh arising from the posterior vulvar area. The vulvar varicosities may be in communication with the LSV, which may be filled from the posterior vulvar veins.

True ovarian varicocele may be diagnosed with ultrasound or phlebography. A congested ovary may be shown by ultrasound, and reflux in the ovarian veins may be observed by color duplex — but only in some patients — during a Valsalva maneuver. The dilated ovarian vein may be demonstrated by direct vulvar venography (Hobbs) or by retrograde phlebography. It is important to exclude other inflammatory conditions (including Crohn's disease, diverticulosis and tumors), vertebral problems causing neural compression as well as genitourinary diseases (ovarian cysts, endometriosis, tumors, etc.).

Localized vulvar veins (particularly in young subjects) may be a separate clinical entity. Cavernosal tissue may also be present. Color and power duplex show the diffuse reticular vascular structure not related to ovarian reflux.

The treatment of PCS may be conservative (suppression of ovarian function) or surgical (retroperitoneal ligation of the veins, oophorectomy or even hysterectomy). Sclerotherapy of the vulvar veins has also been used, using 3% STD, with good results. If untreated, PVC often tends to disappear after the menopause.

25

Lymphatic Diseases

Introduction

In lymphatic channels, there is a continuous flow of lymph — part of the interstitial fluid — including degraded proteins, bacteria and bacterial elements and, generally, residual protein fractions produced by metabolic processes. The fluid constitutes the 2–4 L/d of lymph drained into the subclavian vein and eventually into the systemic circulation. A block or damage of lymphatics or their destruction (e.g., by radiotherapy) impairs lymphatic flow causing distal swelling.

Primary lymphedema (LE) is a definition including idiopathic types of LE with no apparent, clear origin or associated to abnormal lymphatic development, hypoplasia of the lymphatic network and decreased lymphatic diameter or hypotrophy. Congenital LE occurs before 1 year of age, it is often bilateral (more common in males); if the disease is familial, it is defined as "Milroy disease". Primary LE often occurs during adolescence, tends to be unilateral, with a large predominance in females.

LE developing after the age of 35 can be associated to several problems causing obstruction like infections, surgery with removal of lymph nodes, radiotherapy, soft tissue tumors (breast and prostate melanomas tend to spread through local lymphatic channels and, generally, require excision of lymph nodes). With a limited correlation with time, a secondary form of LE may occur in the affected areas. Bacterial and fungal infections, repeated traumas, lymphoproliferative disease are considered less common causes.

(a)

(b)

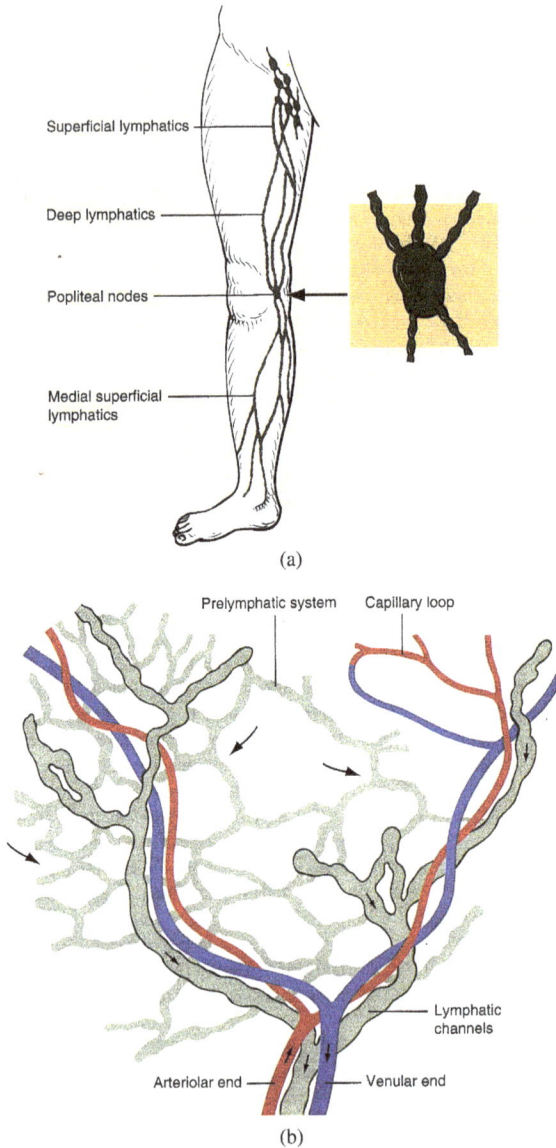

Figure 1. (a) Lymphatic system, lymphatic macrocirculations and microcirculation. (b) The arteriolar end of the system, the venular end and the capillary loop. Prelymphatic spaces are indicated by arrows and drain into the lymphatic channels which follow the course of the artery and vein.

Common parasitic infections can be a major cause of lymphatic obstruction or dilatations (filariasis) with severe forms of LE. It is mainly a tropical infective disease — involving millions — more than a vascular problem. Figure 1 shows the main aspects of the lymphatic system.

Signs/symptoms of LE

The difference in size of the limbs is, generally, visually clear. The limbs present a permanent, painless edema (not receding with elevation of the limb or changing minimally). The difference in limb size is associated in some cases to a history of surgery or radiotherapy. LE associated to parasitic infections may be observed in patients with specific profiles. LE has a slow and painless progression with edema, progressively evolving into tissue fibrosis. The edema is generally nonpitting.

Edema appears more evidently at the dorsum of the foot and at the ankle level. Eventually, dry skin, eczema, hyperkeratosis may appear if the skin is not hydrated and protected. Minor cuts may produce significant infections and mycosis.

Case 1. Radiotherapy. There is no venous component. The limb is "cold".

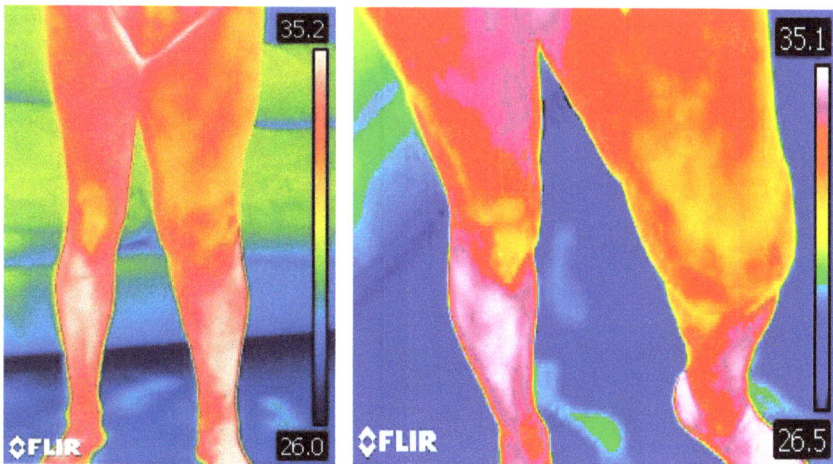

The Angiology Bible

Diagnosis

The diagnosis of LE is usually clear. A difference of >200 mL between the two limbs (e.g., after surgery or irradiation) may be used to define secondary LE. Limb water volumetry is simple, effective and may be used to evaluate progression or the effects of management (Fig. 2).

Ultrasound imaging

Ultrasound shows a concomitant venous involvement (increasing edema) and must always exclude venous obstructions and other venous problems.

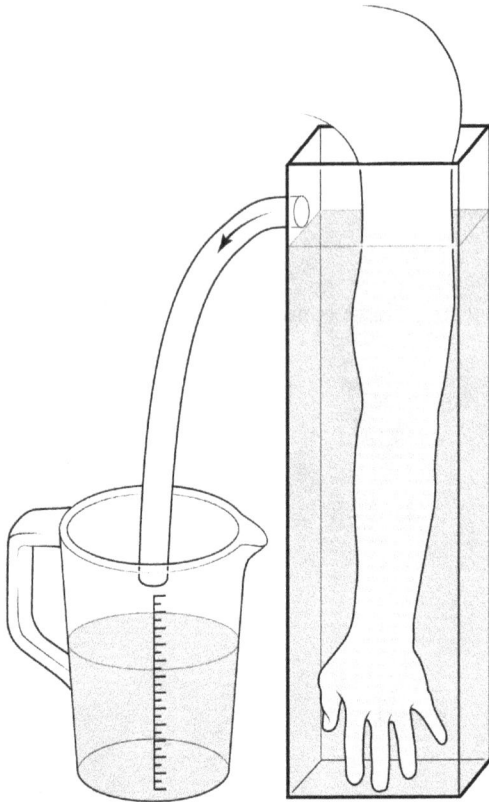

Figure 2. Measurements of arm volume with water displacement. Most lymphatic involvements at the arm are secondary, postsurgical and/or postradiotherapy.

CT and MRI scans are used to exclude the presence of masses or compressions. Lymphangiography is used less now and does not really show the full picture. Often it may further damage the few remaining lymphatic vessels.

Radionuclide lymphoscintigraphy can be considered a standard for evaluating lymphatic function. The test is minimally invasive (^{99m}Tc-labeled dye is injected at the interfinger or intertoe spaces. This procedure has minimal risks of side effects and of damaging the residual vessels. The test gives information of lymphatic flow but the anatomy is not clearly delineated.

Differential diagnosis

Monolateral, permanent swelling is usually lymphatic while bilateral swelling is generally due to systemic causes (kidney disease, hypoproteinemia, heart failure, etc.). Pure lymphatic disease is a rare condition seen in young subjects; most subjects with limb swelling often have a concomitant or associated CVI.

Decreased limb mobility (e.g., in patients with neurological problems) may cause significant monolateral edema. The evaluation of the ratio between plasmatic and interstitial proteins may diagnose edema of lymphatic origin, very early in the clinical evolution (Fig. 3). When interstitial fluid has a protein content superior to the protein content of the plasma, lymphatic involvement is defined.

Treatment of LE

There is no definitive treatment at the moment. The management possibilities are incomplete. Benzopyrones and diuretics may have some efficacy in selected patients.

Therapeutic modalities

Studies with the supplement Robuvit (Horphag), a *Quercus* wood extract, show promising results in primary and secondary LE and also show that

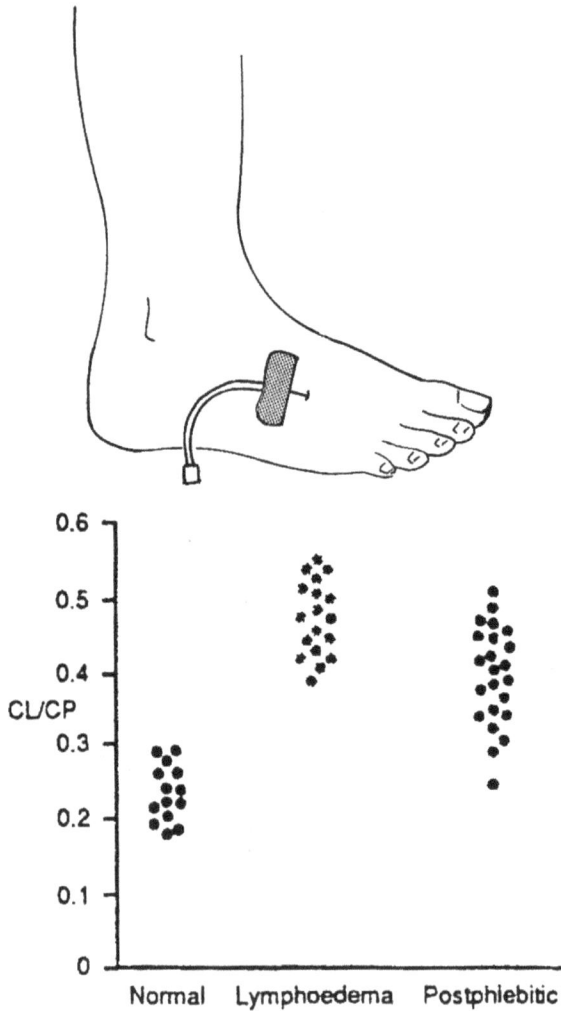

Figure 3.   The ratio between the concentration of interstitial (lymphatic) and plasmatic proteins increases in lymphatic limbs and (less) in chronic venous insufficiency.

the supplement has no side effects. Important levels of elastic compression, selective exercise program, a careful skin care, manual lymphatic drainage or drainage with pneumatic compression and leg elevation offer significant possibilities of improvements on a very individual basis.

Decongestive lymphatic therapy (DLT) includes a management with lymph drainage, compression, intermittent compression and exercise. It is important to avoid dry skin and even minor breaks, infections and cuts. Any infection is more difficult to heal as normal lymphatics drain bacteria into the lymphatic system creating a response defense mechanism, absent or impaired in these patients.

Surgical treatment

Surgical treatment of LE is considered in a rare case: it includes debulking, liposuction of the excess in subcutaneous tissues, reconstructive methods with removal of fat and skin and the fibrotic areas, when possible. Lipectomy for the upper arm includes fat and subcutaneous tissues removal with restoration of the normal volume of the limb.

In some patients, lymphatic channels may be reconstructed with lymphovenous anastomoses when the dilated lymphatics are suitable (Fig. 4). However, distal fibrosis after these procedures does not seem to change with surgery.

Transplantation

Transplantation of lymphatic tissue has been used in selected subjects. The lymph nodes are harvested from a healthy inguinal space (or from the axillary space) and can be reimplanted and may develop new lymphatic channels (Fig. 5).

The harvested lymphatic tissue can be sectioned in small parts that are implanted into the affected limbs on the basis of the LE distribution (for instance, along the LSV). The implanted parts tend to grow lymphatic channels in time improving lymphatic outflow. The procedure is minimally invasive and can be made under local anesthetic (Fig. 6).

An evolution of this procedure consists in harvesting lymphatic tissue, regrowing cells in culture. The cells can be reimplanted with repeated injections (Fig. 7). The lymph tissue probably has significant direct vasogenic properties creating new channels in areas where there is a limited or altered lymphatic network.

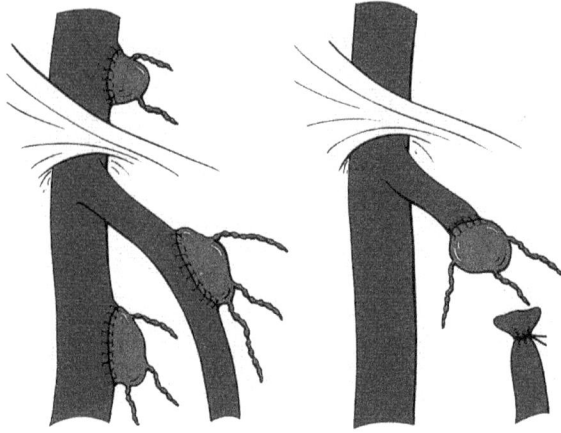

Figure 4.   Different types of lymphovenous anastomosis have been attempted with variable success when lymphatics are enlarged and usable.

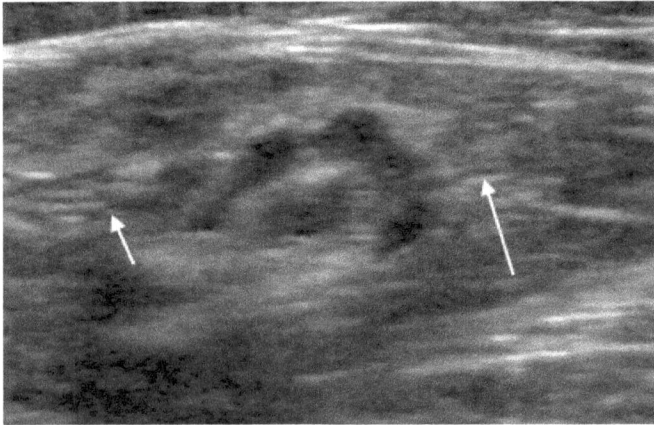

Figure 5.   A transplanted lymph node develops in some 12 months new lymphatic channels that may make connections with the local native system.

A high-resolution ultrasound image shows new lymphatic channels (arrows) appearing from a transplanted small lymph node, 12 months after the implant. The technology of lymphatic transplant needs evolution but the problem is relatively rare and solutions may constitute a marginal "market" with a limited commercial interest.

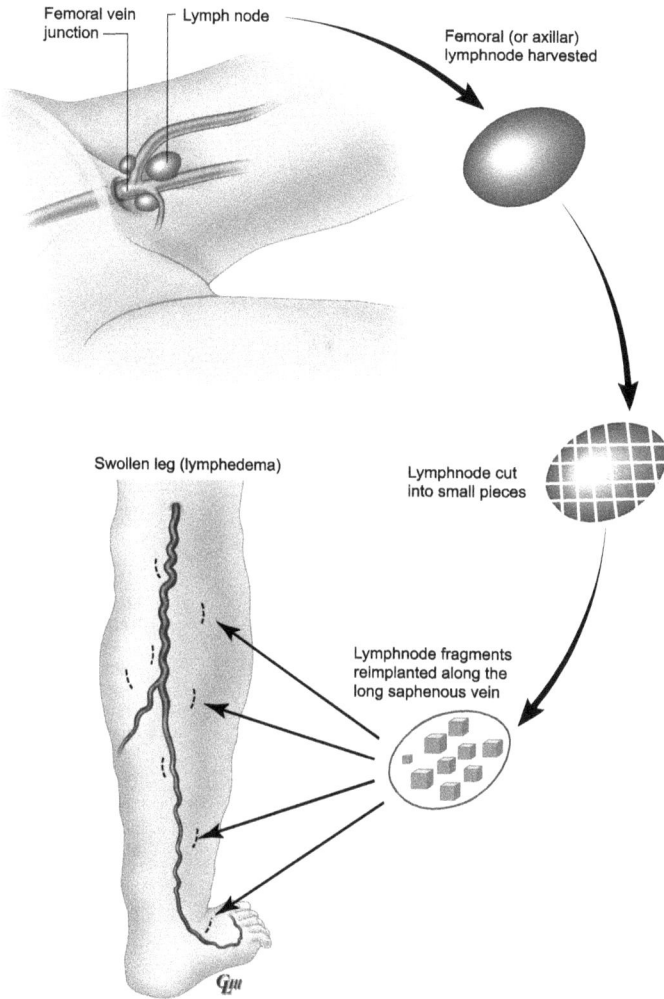

Figure 6.   The diagram of the original study on lymphatic transplant. Lymphatic tissue is harvested, made into small parts and reimplanted along the LSV. The intervention can be made under local anesthesia.

Complications of LE

In time, swelling may be massive and the limb may become unusable. Ulcerations and infections may be repeated. A lymphangiosarcoma or angiosarcoma may rarely arise from chronic lymphedematous limbs. This neoplastic transformation is defined as Stewart–Treves syndrome.

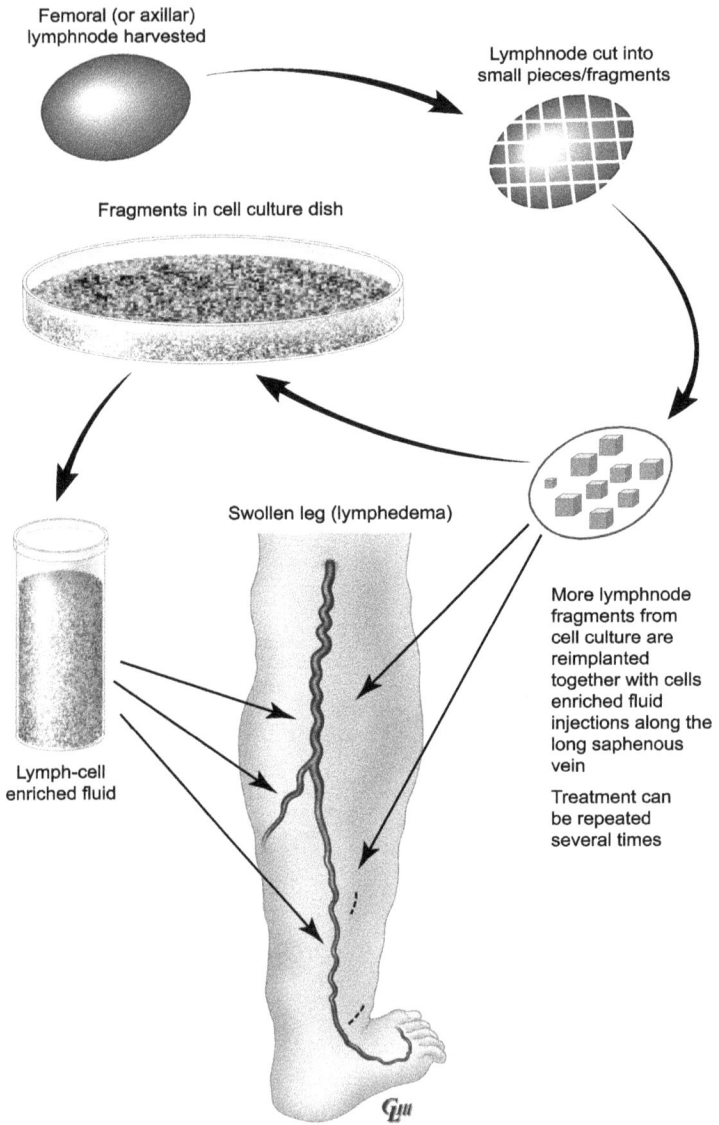

Femoral (or axillar)
lymphnode harvested

Lymphnode cut into
small pieces/fragments

Fragments in cell culture dish

Swollen leg (lymphedema)

More lymphnode
fragments from
cell culture are
reimplanted
together with cells
enriched fluid
injections along the
long saphenous
vein

Treatment can
be repeated
several times

Lymph-cell
enriched fluid

Figure 7.　Variation of the lymphatic transplant. Lymphatic tissue is harvested, made into small parts and grown in cell cultures. The grown lymphatic cells are periodically reimplanted with injections along the LSV.

26

Analects, Fragments and Angiological Tips

Carotid stories

Plaque factors

The complex, dyshomogeneous and low-density carotid plaque with a thrombogenic, irregular plaque-luminal interface is shown in the following figure.

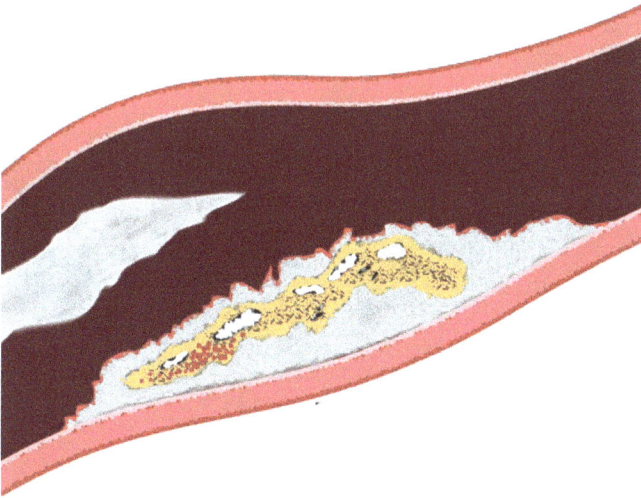

When evaluating carotid plaques (by high-resolution ultrasound), stenosis is an important "flow" factor but other aspects are essential. The surface of the plaque must be considered (a more irregular surface promotes thrombus formation and platelet adhesion and consequent embolization). The homogenicity of the core structure with minimal differences in density is associated to a clinically less dangerous plaque.

On ultrasound, low-density areas (i.e., clots, liquified lipids) have a very low echogenicity while fibrotic plaques (including more collagen and elastin) are more echogenic and stable. Lower density, dyshomogeneity, different layers of thrombotic appositions, surface irregularities all contribute to a lower plaque stability and to its more dangerous behavior.

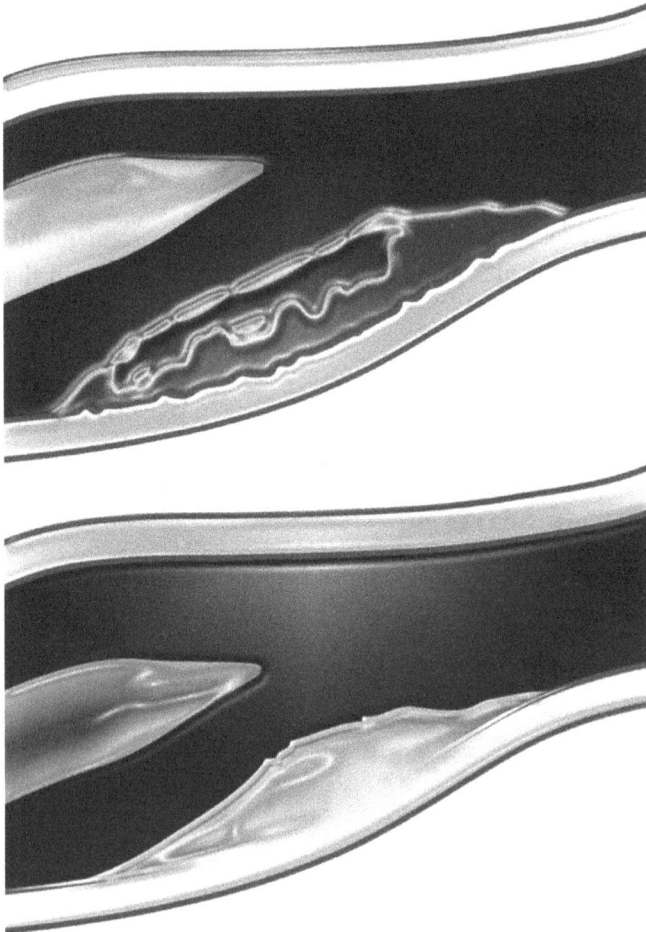

Making the plaque more stable and more echogenic is possible using natural products (pharma-standard supplements) that modulate the production of collagen. Arterial plaques are basically keloids: irregular, disorganized growths/scarrings in response (out of proportion) to an initial arterial injury. The regularization of the scarring, resulting in a more echogenic and stable plaque (as seen in the following figure), has been obtained in selected patients using the combination Pycnogenol–*Centella asiatica*. Pycnogenol is a powerful antioxidant and anti-inflammatory natural agent; *Centella asiatica* is a natural modulator of collagen growth. Several studies indicate that plaques can be made safer and stable, independently from risk factor management.

The above figure shows the evolution of an irregular carotid plaque with mixed and low echogenicity into a more "fibrotic", echogenic, stable plaque with a more regular plaque-lumen interface, less prone to thrombosis and embolization. The level of greyscale median increases with an increase in density (white parts in the schematic image, as seen by ultrasound).

Flow factors

In many patients with carotid and vertebral symptoms, plaques are not the only cause of symptoms. A decrease in intervertebral spaces with a thinner disk makes the cervical column shorter, and the carotid and vertebral become tortuous and irregular. Neck motion can further alter the flow by making the arteries temporarily even more curvy and irregular. Straightening the neck with a simple, soft collar can extend the cervical column by some 3–4 cm in months. The straightened arteries bring flow better into the brain and many "flow" symptoms tend to disappear.

In some older subjects with neck shortening, a simple noninvasive management like this may solve some problems and even prevent a number of TIAs and strokes. The relative stenosis value of the most important plaques is decreased when the artery is more rectilinear and stream friendly with a better internal flow dynamic and decreased shear stress.

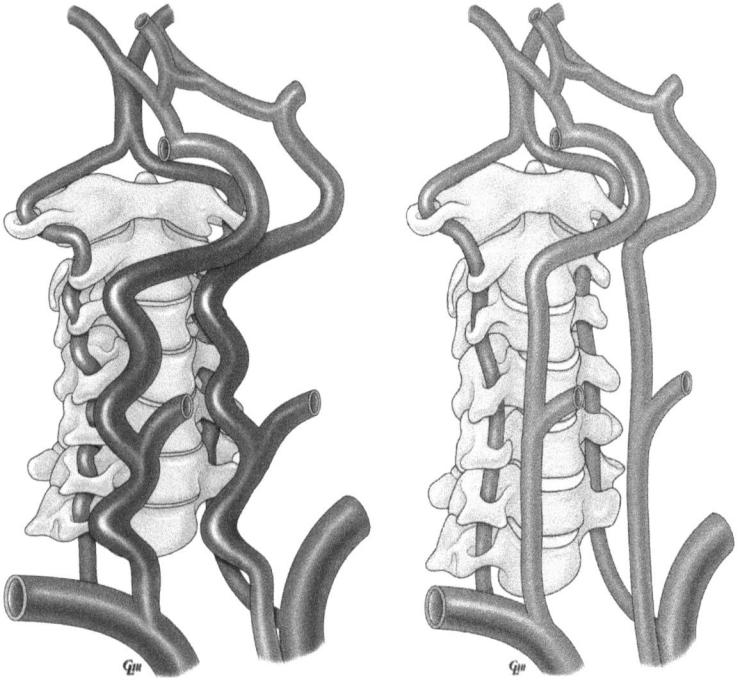

Plaque "tectonics"

As in geological plaque tectonics, there is an initial fragmentation of the intima–media complex seen as a discontinuity in the linear arterial patterns. The following figure shows another example of fragmentation of the IMT wafer.

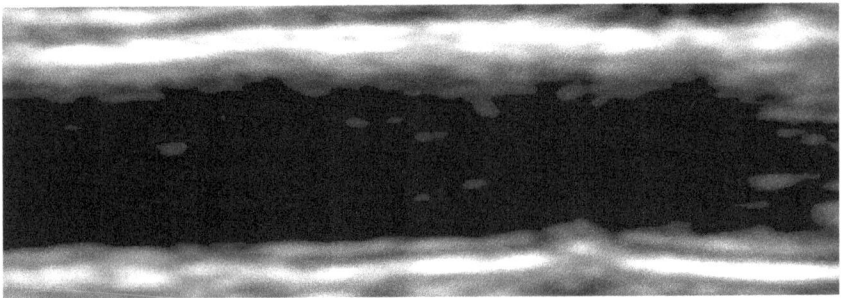

Part of the fragment goes below the IMT layers a start proliferating pushing toward the lumen (up) the IMT layers above it.

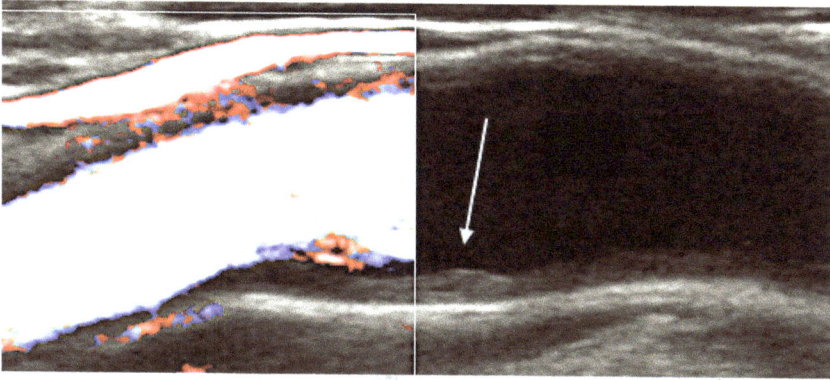

The subduction part of the plaque goes deep and the upper, internal, extrusional or luminal part goes up, often impacting the luminal flow more directly and presenting a thrombogenic surface.

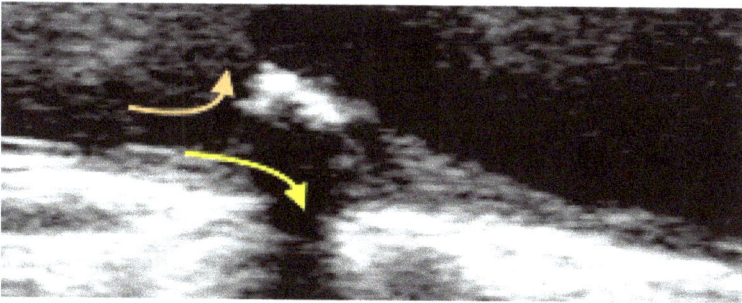

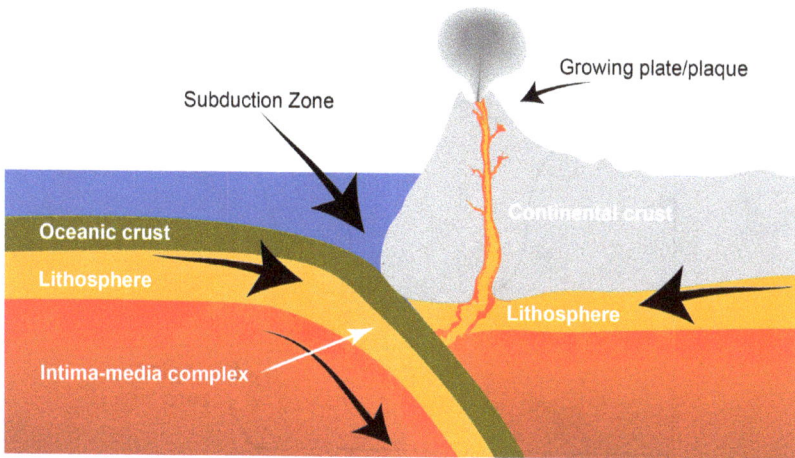

Subductional and extrusional part of the plaque may have a different destiny. If the extrusion is against the flow, it may easily break, embolize, cause clots and dynamic flow alterations or even a (partial) dissection.

Plaque "tectonics" is visible with high-resolution ultrasound in most plaques in evolution, without calcifications.

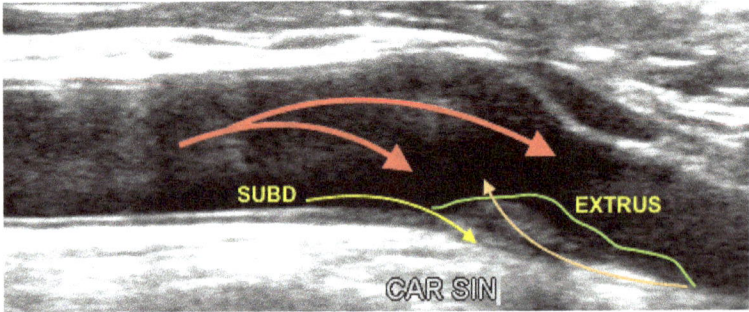

Microcirculation tips

There are different methods to assess the microcirculation. There is no vascular medicine of angiology without mastering microcirculatory methods.

All measurements are made in a room at controlled temperature (i.e., 22°C). Laser Doppler (LD) flowmetry (or fluxmetry) is the most practical method. Occluding the arterial circulation, there is still a signal due to Newtonian motion in the sample volume. This quota is not "real" flow and should be eliminated from the final number. Most LD flowmeters have options to regulate this factor.

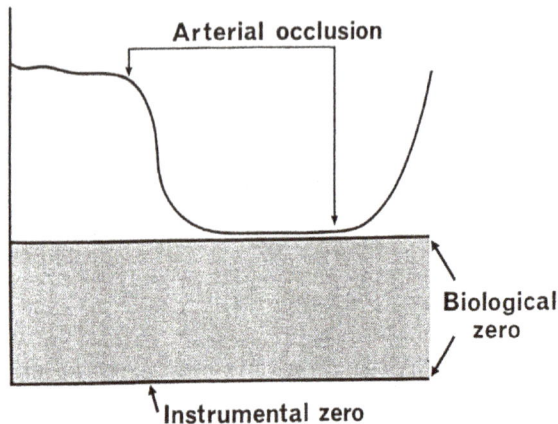

The measurements of flux is basically a factor — a stochastic representation — deriving from the number of red blood cells in the sample volume multiplied by their velocity. It is possible to have a high output with a high number of cells moving slowly or a minor number of cells moving faster. The flux "number" is not parametric and needs interpretation. Part of the flux we measure is thermoregularory flux that would not affect, for instance, nutrition and healing. The real nutritional flow — what we need to increase in case of ischemia — is a limited part. In this nutritional layer, flux and O_2 have parallel distributions. The use of special polycarbonate spacers allow to detect a signal with a predominant nutritional component.

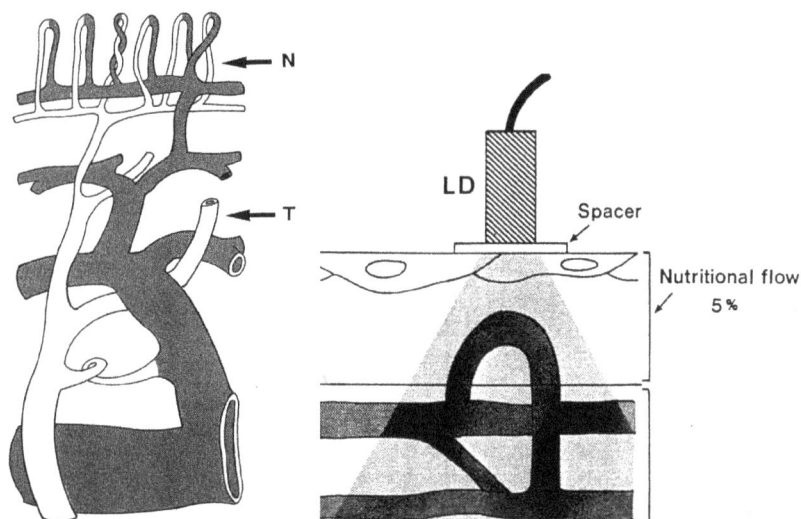

In fingers and distal skin — strictly humans — the capillary and nutritional flow and flux are corresponding in some measurements and must be considered for clinical evaluation. Changes in the thermoregulatory flow do not improve or alter healing. Each LD has its own measurements.

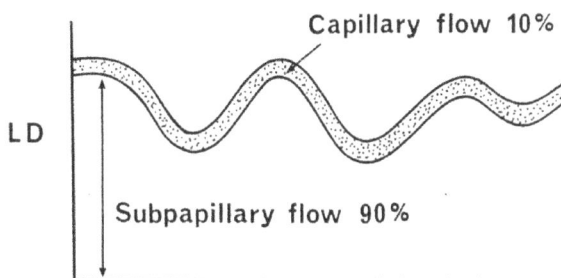

Capillary filtration (CF) can be measured in mL/min in 100 cc of tissue with strain-gauge plethysmography. A 23 cm cuff is placed and the arteries and veins are occluded (i.e., for 10 min). After a period of venous dilatation, increase in volume and distension of the system, there is a plateau that shows a very minimal and slow increase. The tangent to the curve between 7 and 10 min is considered a measurement of CF.

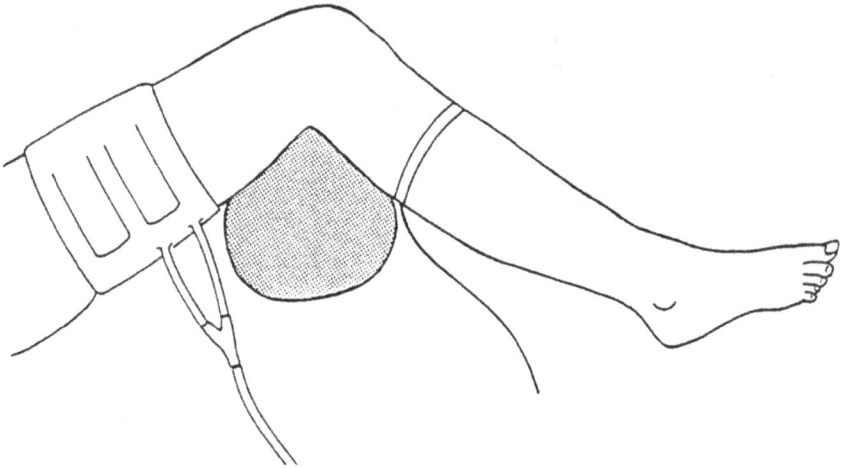

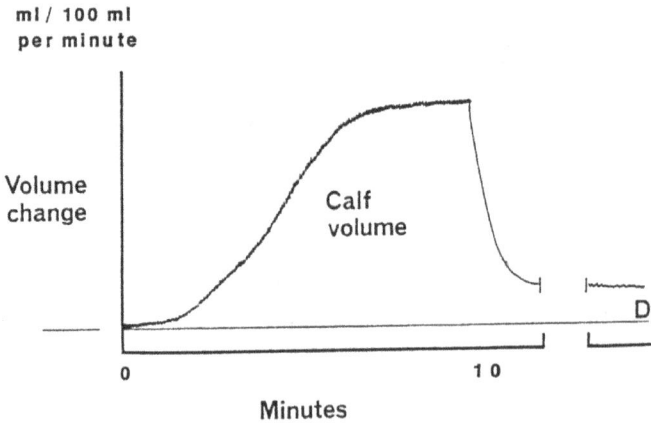

In venous disease in diabetes and in many clinical problems associated to edema and swelling, CF increased. The method is mainly used to assess treatments. CF can also be measured asking the patient to stand and measuring the accumulation of interstitial fluid in an established time (rate of ankle swelling).

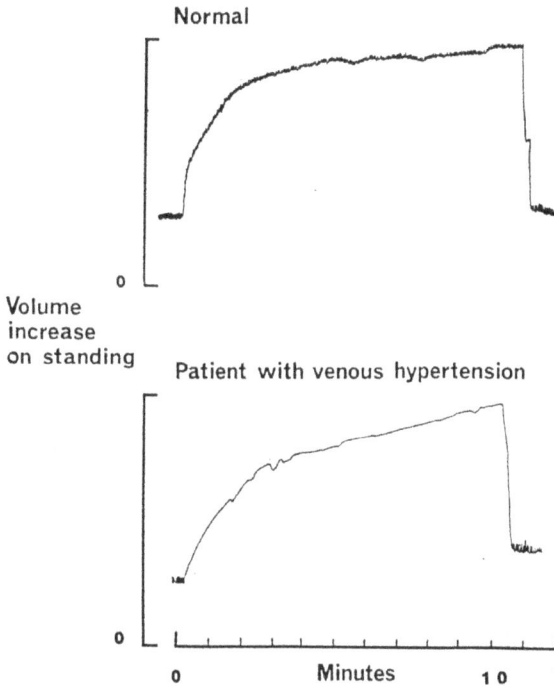

Strain gauges also allow measurements of perfusion pressure (i.e., toes) when a Doppler signal is too weak to be recorded. In venous disease, there is a good correlation in chronic venous hypertension between ambulatory venous pressure (vertical axis in mmHg) and distal, perimalleolar flux at rest.

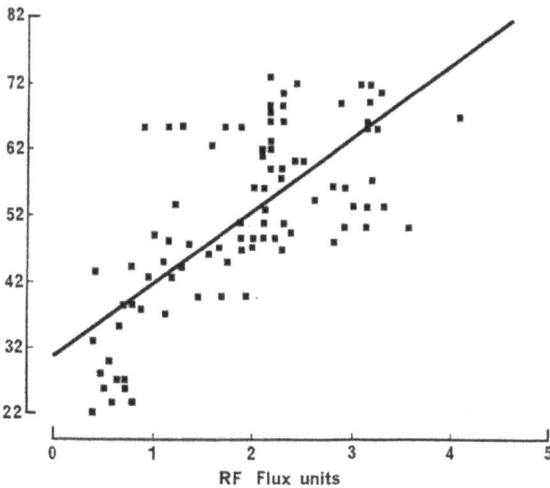

Interesting measurements can be made in diabetic microangiopathy with LD. Microangiopathic alterations may be present years before arterial flow alterations and skin lesions are visible or measurable. Both venous and diabetic microangiopathies are characterized by high flux levels and can be defined as high-perfusion microangiopathies. Microcirculatory measurements in animals have a very minimal correspondence with human microcirculation.

3D vascular imaging

3D imaging from CT scans or MRI enables early diagnosis and makes pretreatment evaluation more targeted. Programs like Osirix now are a routine part of any vascular investigation.

These evaluations are very effective for controls after surgery or interventional methods.

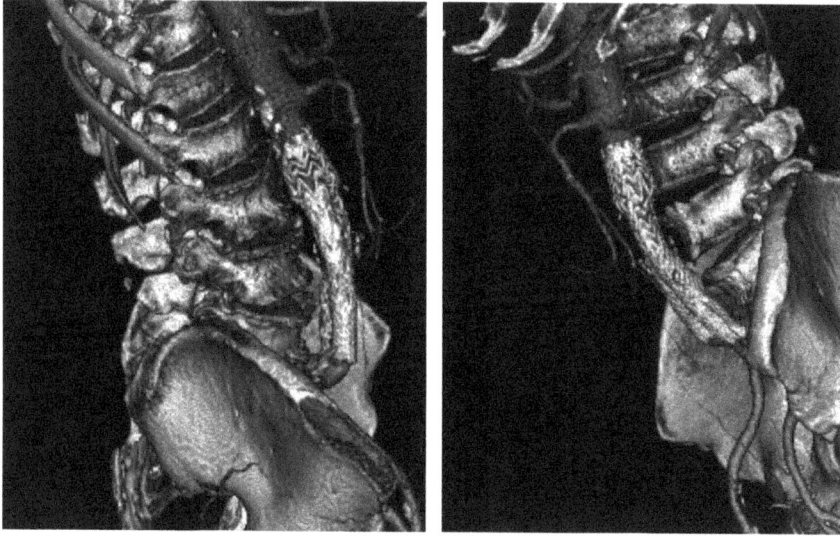

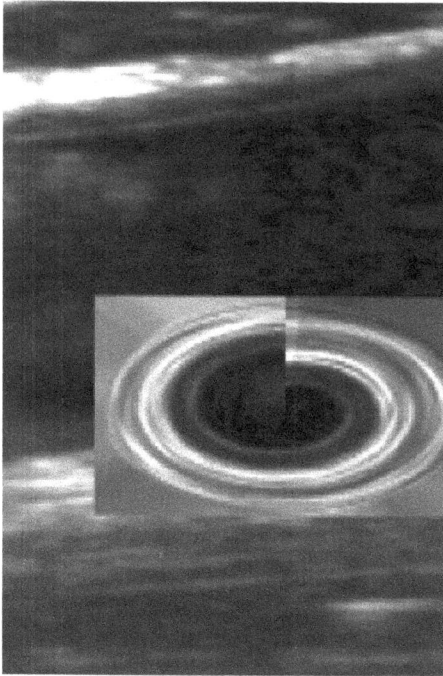

Early preclinical atherosclerosis.

Reconstruction of the intima–media thickening seen in an anticlockwise circular pattern from serial samples of the same artery in 3 years in subjects with very high risk level. The increase in thickness of the arterial wall is visible and the increase in the size of the layers — at the beginning and end of the observation period — is an indicator of intima–media thickness (IMT) growth rate in this image. Thickening is different from plaque morphology. In thickening, the layers are thicker but we can recognize them. In plaques, the layers are not recognizable anymore. The wafer structure is lost.

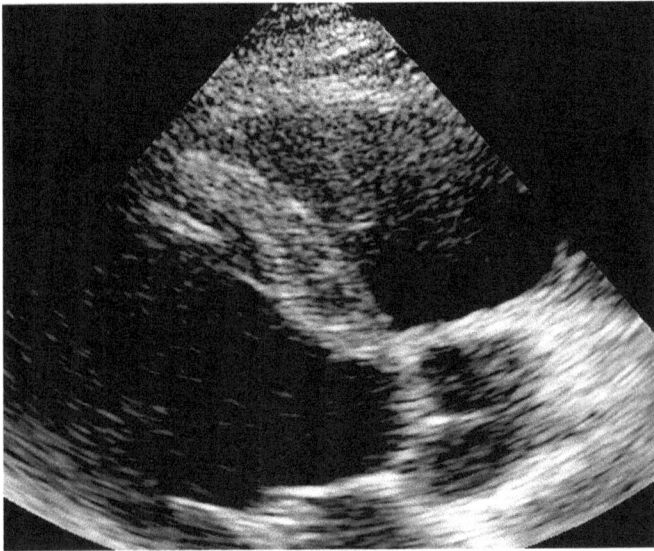

Always look at the heart.

In all vascular patients, it is imperative, during the vascular examination with ultrasounds, to evaluate the heart. Left ventricular function, coronary calcifications, enlargement of the chambers, etc. are generally visible in minutes in a preliminary evaluation. Specific findings may be better evaluated by a cardiologist.

IMT evaluation is now easy and reproducible. IMT evaluation is a general evaluation af all the cardiovascular risk factors. It is more effective as a population evaluation than as an individual measurement. It is not possible in most ultrasound images to separate the intima from the media.

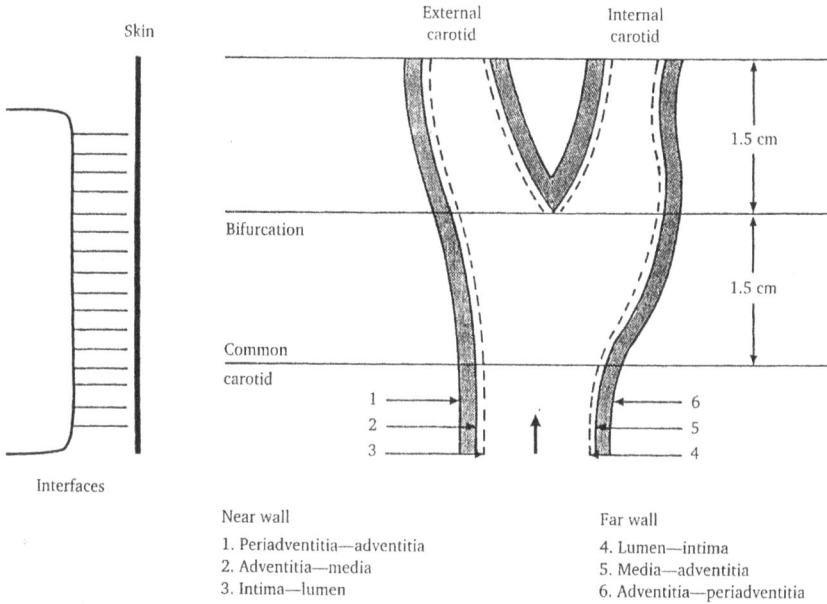

The IMT at the carotid. In any population, there are defined values for thickness according to age.

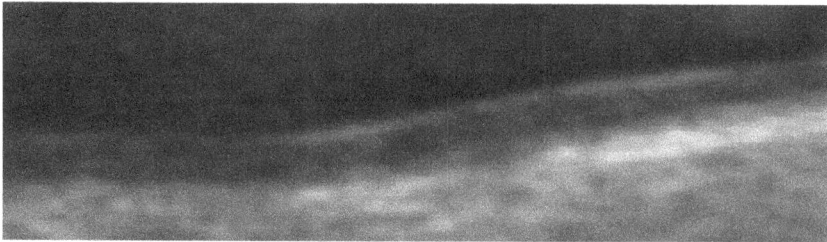

Screening

The main problem and challenge in cardiovascular disease is population screening which may reveal thickness, plaques and other alterations (i.e., aneurysms) years before clinical problems. The healthcare systems can just cope with patients with clinical conditions. Preclinical alterations evaluation and cardiovascular screening should be organized and made by communities more than healthcare providers. Population screening is cost effective and reveals the segment of population with that specific problem allowing to plan community interventions. The result of screening is a *screened-out population*, without problems. For the part of population with problems, specific interventions can be planned.

The unhealthy philosophy of screening is the aim of catching subjects with minimal problems transforming them into "productive" patients in supposed need of treatments and new tests. Specific screening plans may be needed in different populations according to the presence of diseases.[1]

PGE1

Treatment of peripheral vascular disease with PGE1 is possibly the main direct, vascular medical intervention useful to improve perfusion and control signs/symptoms due to ischemia. Focusing on the easiest prostaglandin, PGE1, the treatment can be administered without significant side effects to almost all vascular patients at low costs and without the need for hospital admission or complex monitoring.

Medical treatments support interventional treatments and surgery and cannot be considered competitive to interventional methods. The medical aspects need to be blended with interventional methods all the time. A "standard" infusion of PGE1 (i.e., 60 μg in 50–100 mL of saline in 30 min) improves claudication, signs/symptoms in critical limb ischemia and may help limit the amputation levels in most patients.

PGE1 has significant activities on other organs also, improving cardiac, kidney and cerebral perfusion at the same time.

The low cost of prostaglandin (PGE1) and its expired patent are its main weak points: compensations for a PGE1 infusion tend to be very low; therefore, institutions and physicians tend to focus on more profitable treatments/managements like catheter intervention or amputations. Regular PGE1 treatment appears to decrease the amputation rate and

---

[1] See *Vascular Screening* by G. Belcaro, A. N. Nicolaides and M. Veller (Edizioni Minerva Medica).

global survival in most vascular patients with severe claudication and critical limb ischemia.

This study is still in progress (in the graph, PGX = PGE1) with specific attention to costs.

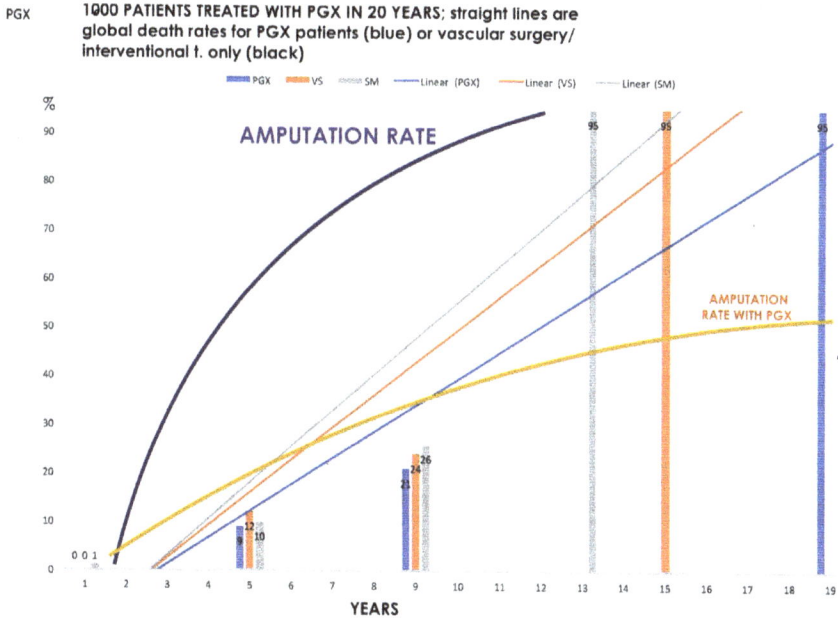

PGX 1000 PATIENTS TREATED WITH PGX IN 20 YEARS; straight lines are global death rates for PGX patients (blue) or vascular surgery/interventional t. only (black)

Antiplatelet agents or antiaggregants (AAs)

AAs include the following:

- Irreversible cyclooxygenase (COX) inhibitors
  - Aspirin
  - Triflusal (Disgren)
- Adenosine diphosphate (ADP) receptor inhibitors
  - Clopidogrel (Plavix)
  - Prasugrel (Effient)
  - Ticagrelor (Brilinta)
  - Ticlopidine (Ticlid)

- Phosphodiesterase inhibitors
  o Cilostazol (Pletal)
- Protease-activated receptor-1 (PAR-1) antagonists
  o Vorapaxar (Zontivity)
- Glycoprotein IIb/IIIa inhibitors (intravenous use only)
  o Abciximab (ReoPro)
  o Eptifibatide (Integrilin)
  o Tirofiban (Aggrastat)
- Adenosine reuptake inhibitors
  o Dipyridamole (Persantine)
- Thromboxane inhibitors
  o Thromboxane synthase inhibitors
  o Thromboxane receptor antagonists
  o Terutroban

AAs decrease platelet aggregation and inhibit thrombus formation, generally, in the arterial circulation, where anticoagulants have limited effects. AAs are used in prevention of thrombotic and embolizing cerebrovascular or cardiovascular disease. AAs interfere with platelet activation (primary hemostasis).

AAs reversibly or irreversibly inhibit the process involved in platelet activation resulting in decreased tendency of platelets to adhere to one another, to thrombogenic surfaces or agents including normal and altered endothelium. Aspirin generally increases the risk of bleeding. One subject in 800 per year may have a bleeding problem due to low-dose aspirin. *Dual antiplatelet therapy* is also used to obtain greater antiplatelet activity when needed. *Prevention of arterial thrombosis* is considered essential in patients with conditions at risk of thromboembolism. AAs are used to prevent stroke, in atrial fibrillation, after heart surgery (especially prosthetic valves), angina, unstable angina in subjects with coronary stent, arterial disease and apical/ventricular/mural thrombus. *Aspirin* and *Triflusal* inhibit COX, reducing platelet production of thromboxane A_2 (TXA_2, a powerful vasoconstrictor that lowers cyclic adenosine monophosphate (AMP) and initiates the platelet release reaction). *Dipyridamole* inhibits platelet phosphodiesterase and increases cyclic AMP with potentiation of the action of

PGI_2, opposing the actions of TXA_2. *Clopidogrel* mainly affects ADP-dependent activation of IIb/IIIa complex.

Glycoprotein IIb/IIIa receptor antagonists block receptors on platelets used for fibrinogen and von Willebrand factor. Following are few examples of these antagonists:

- Synthetic nonpeptides (e.g., tirofiban)
- Murine–human chimeric antibodies (e.g., abciximab)
- Synthetic peptides (e.g., eptifibatide)

Epoprostenol is a prostacyclin used to inhibit aggregation during renal dialysis (with or without heparin) and is also used in primary pulmonary hypertension.

AAs have *important side effects* that must be considered. Drug toxicity may be increased when multiple antiplatelet drugs are used. Gastrointestinal problems, including bleeding, are common adverse events (particularly for Aspirin) seen in many patients.

AAs are an indispensable part of vascular medicine — as anticoagulants — and a complete, specific knowledge must be acquired to manage vascular conditions.

Plaques in penile fibrosis

Penile plaques are considered a cheloidal scarring process, comparable to plaques in the arterial system. The composition of the plaques and their evolution — including calcifications — are comparable if not parallel. These plaques do not respond effectively to the effects of risk factor control management (hypertension, lipid control). Higher oxidative stress may be a significant factor in the evolution of these plaques.

These cheloids are produced, usually as a response to even minimal trauma (i.e., catheters) and respond to management with *Centella asiatica*, the only modulator of collagen and elastin. This product has a natural origin and it is also active on plaques evolution. Generally, penile flow in subjects with these plaques is good. In the following image, a penile plaque produces an acoustic shadow due to calcification.

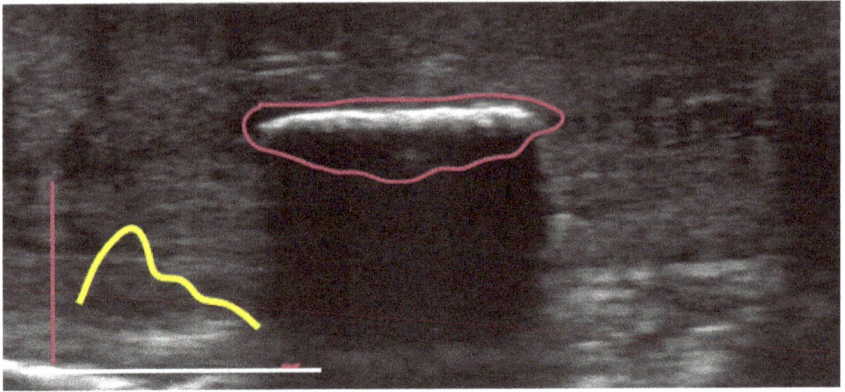

Elastosonography shows the density of the tissue and plaque elements.

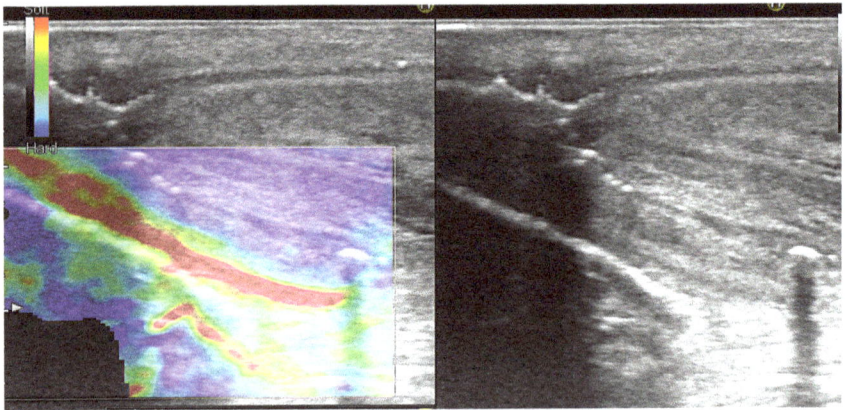

Valvuloplasty

In dilated veins (as in this popliteal vein), the cusps become incompetent. A direct suture on the vein (yellow line) can make the valve cusps (just visible through the vein wall and underlined by white lines) closer and competent again. In postthrombotic limbs, the destruction of the popliteal valves with recanalization makes this type of surgery almost impossible. A valvulated vein segment can be transplanted.

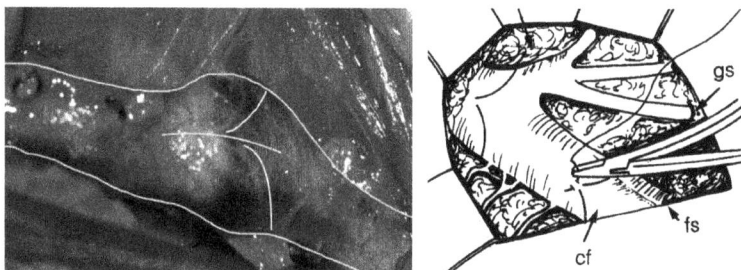

Courtesy of D. Christopoulos and A. N. Nicolaides.

The common femoral vein can also be made competent by restricting the lumen with a fine suture; in the image, instruments and needle (and the surgical exposure) are bigger than real. Limited anterior valvuloplasty (LAP) is made without fully dissecting the vein. Complete dissection of these veins destroys the vasa vasorum network and exposes to dilatation the treated segment. A "full" valvuloplasty requires complete dissection of the vein. An external "net" is usually needed as a protection against dilatation.

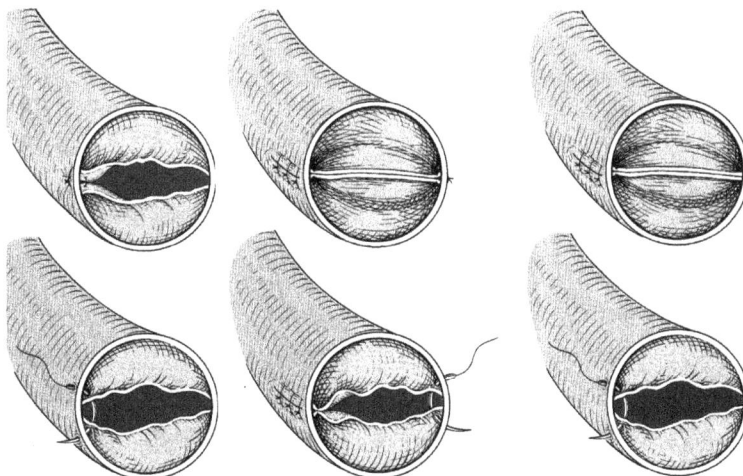

Sclerotherapy

It is the easiest and most cost-effective method of treating VV. It is not perfect, but in combination with selective surgery, it may be a low-cost treatment for patients anywhere in the world. Sclerotherapy is surgery and needs surgical training.

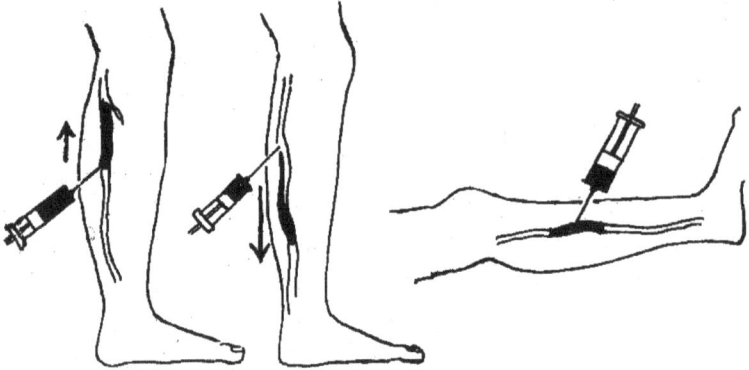

Source: Image from Kimmonnth JB, Robertson DJ (St. Barth's Hospital, London), the *Year Book of Surgery 1949*, "Injection and treatment of varicose veins" (*Br J Surg*, Jan 1949).

Our group has produced the first book on foam sclerotherapy.[2] At the moment, standard sclerotherapy appears to be more selective and effective than foam sclerotherapy which can be used for selected cases. The production of foam is still not standardized and has produced central embolizations.

Minimally invasive methods

A combination of selective surgery and sclerotherapy is possbile with the precise indications of noninvasive tests, particularly ultrasound. There is no need, in most cases, for destructive surgery. Competent or

---

[2] See *Sclerotherapy in Venous Disease* by G. Belcaro, G. Geroulakos, M. R. Cesarone and A. N. Nicolaides (Edizioni Minerva Medica).

dilated vein segments can be made competent again with minimal interventions.

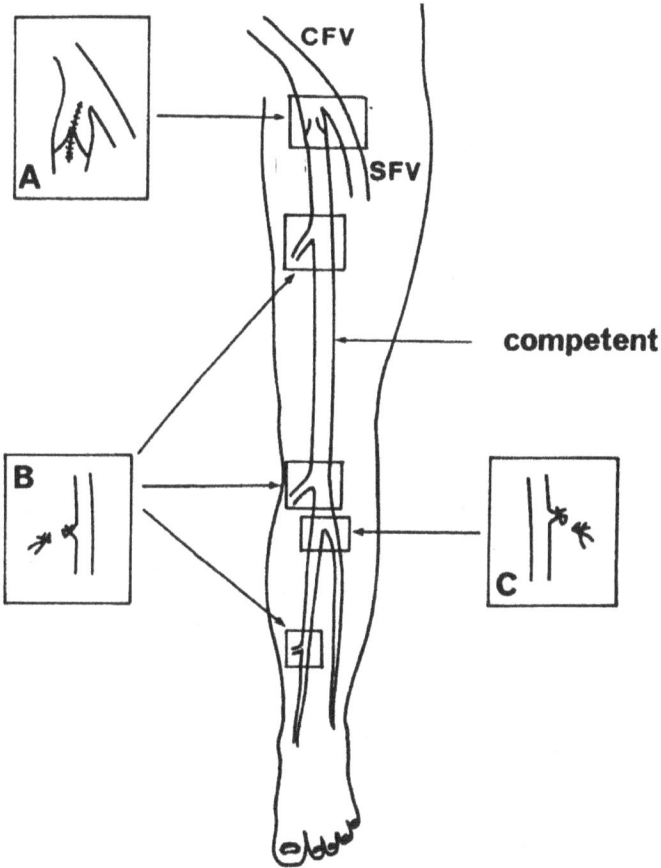

Note: CFV — common femoral vein, SFV — superficial femoral vein, A, B, C — selective surgical treatments.

The closed loop

Ligation of a vein loop without exposure of the endothelium (as seen in the direct section of the veins) may reduce the development of new, recurrent veins and revascularization in the surgical area. The endothelial surface has been considered a significant prorevascularization factor after surgery.

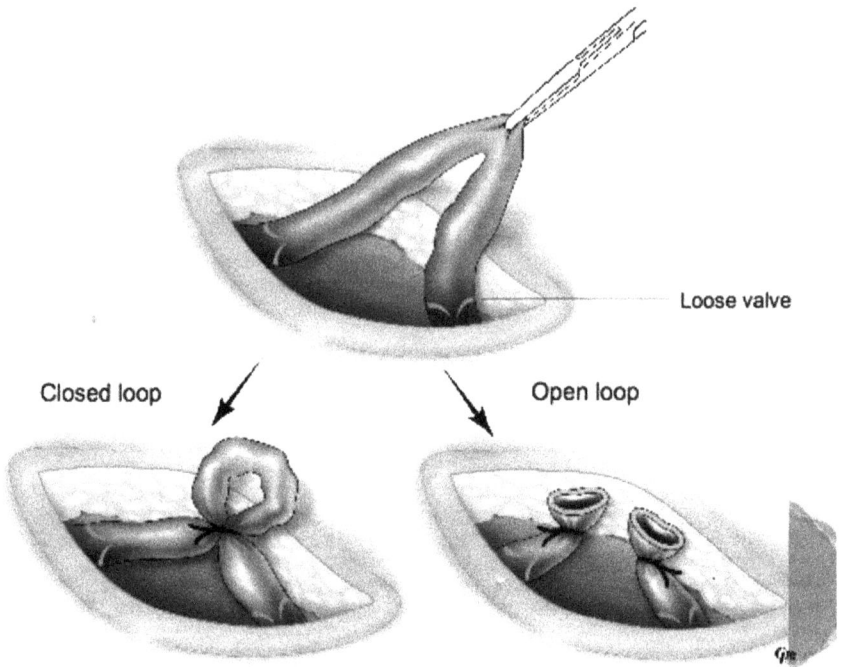

Small vascular networks and minimal "strokes"

Retinal flow

The retinal circulation and flow are part of cerebral flow; an evaluation by ultrasound is an evaluation and an expression of the conditions of cerebral perfusion (including the presence of vasospastic conditions). Ischemic vascular conditions in the eye and optic nerve endings (and the circle of Zinn–Haller, as seen in the ultrasound image) are associated to a large number of problems that require a vascular evaluation including glaucoma. Many episodes of sudden loss of vision (SLV) are associated to acute ischemic/thrombotic conditions. They are real strokes. Retinal thrombois is a common event and, in time, improvements can be observed in most patients. Arterial retinal occlusion and thrombosis lead to acute and more permanent damages. Diabetic retinopathy is a very common condition in search of a better definition, understanding and management methods.

Retinal thrombosis is possibly related to specific risk factors (i.e., the shape of the eye), different from the risk factors found in DVT and to the general concepts of thrombophilia. Heparin and antiplatelet agents seem to be relatively ineffective and may produce bleeding. In general, retinal circulation is a very important sector that needs more attention in circulation sciences as it is not only limited to ophthalmological problems but it is also an expression of significant vascular conditions.

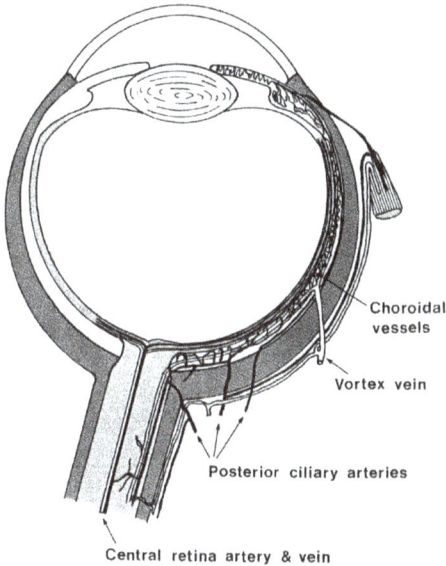

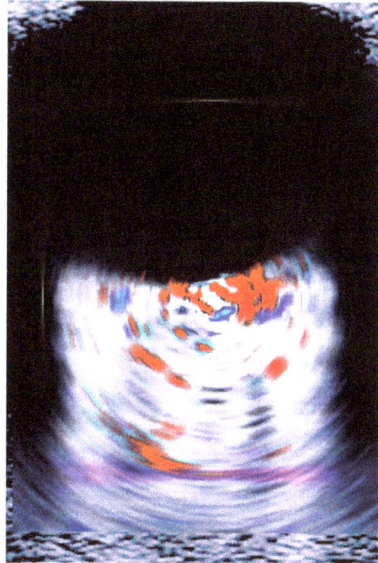

Cochlear circulation

Cochlear circulation is a small, terminal network comparable to the retinal circulation. This cerebral extrusion and alterations in flow/perfusion in a small, limited space without lymphatic drainage have significant effects (loss of hearing, tinnirus, vertigo). Flow can be measured by ultrasound in some patients with an acoustic window or can be evaluated by MRI.

Flow alterations may produce an infarction (with loss of hearing), variable symptoms (physiologically comparable to angina) and strokes with permanent damage to the delicate cells.

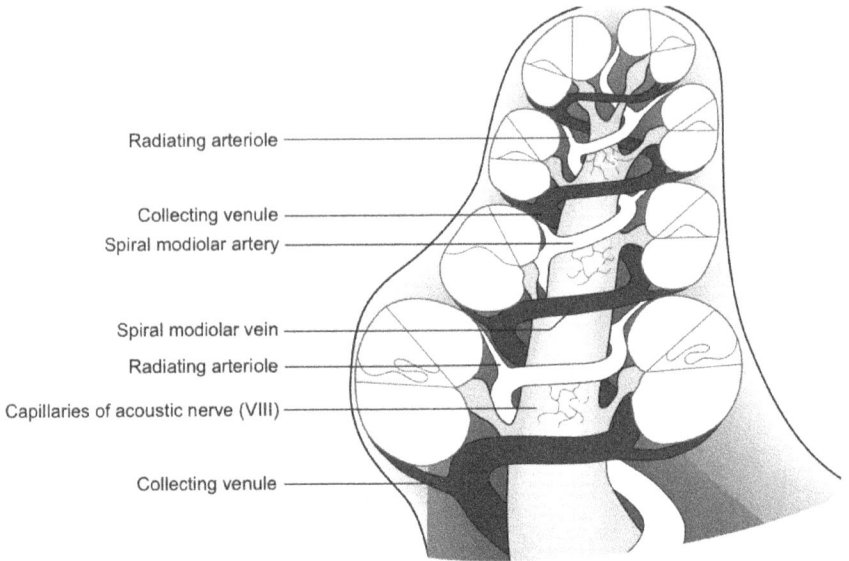

Radiating arteriole

Collecting venule
Spiral modiolar artery

Spiral modiolar vein
Radiating arteriole
Capillaries of acoustic nerve (VIII)

Collecting venule

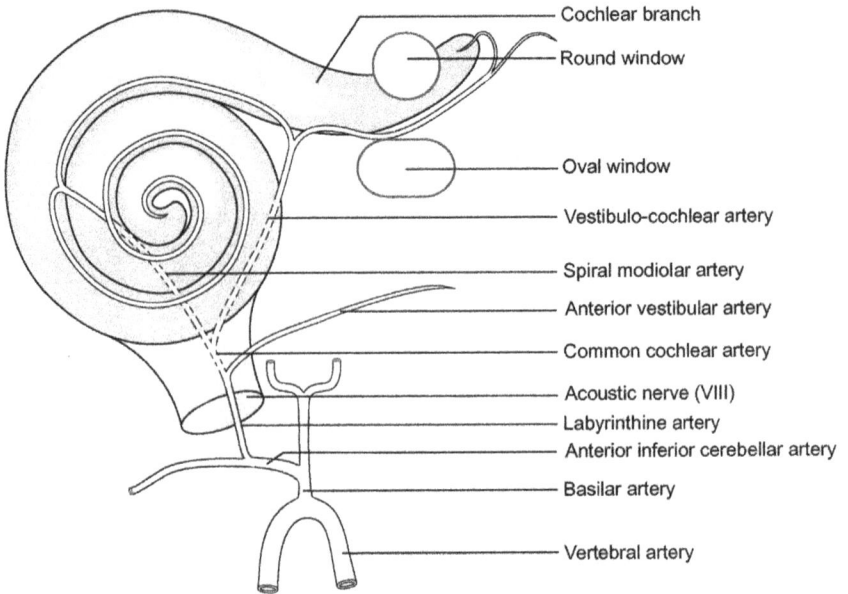

Cochlear branch
Round window
Oval window
Vestibulo-cochlear artery
Spiral modiolar artery
Anterior vestibular artery
Common cochlear artery
Acoustic nerve (VIII)
Labyrinthine artery
Anterior inferior cerebellar artery
Basilar artery
Vertebral artery

These "minimal strokes" at retinal and cochlear levels can be treated in many patients and perfusion can be restored when possible, i.e., with PGE1 infusions. The patients are usually able to detect clearly and soon the effects of treatments.

This terminal, minicirculatory network has a very interesting anatomical design and can be affected as a target organ (i.e., by endothelial dysfunction), years before symptoms can be observed in other parts of the vascular system.

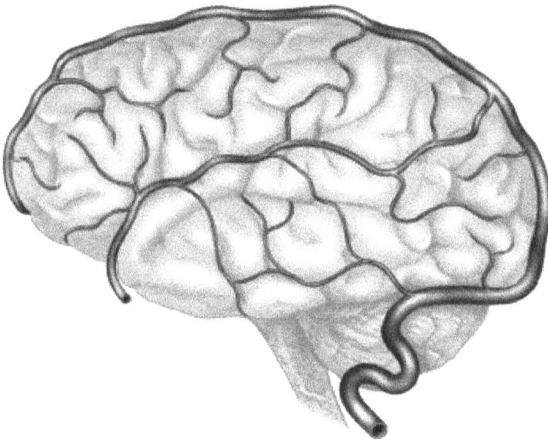

Cerebral vein thrombosis (CVT)

This vascular entity is still an unclear cluster of conditions leading to thrombosis of cerebral veins. CVT may be observed in adults and children and may cause cerebral infarction.

Symptoms are associated with the distribution of the affected veins. Most signs/symptoms are very variable: in children, disidratation and sudden headache may be observed. Headache after using oral contraceptives or sudden, unexplained convulsions can be seen in women. A comatose status with dilated pupils may be another sign. Infections and immunological conditions may be involved. Neuronal ischemia and petechial hemorrhages may be present. Cerebral edema follows vein dilatation.

Cytotoxic edema or vasogenic edema with alterations of the blood–brain barrier may also be seen in CVT. Edema may regress with treatment. Thrombotic occlusions of major sinuses cause intracranic hypertension and altered liquor reabsorption. Usually no dilatation of cerebral ventricular spaces is observed. Causes may be different and often obscure: direct causes, trauma during delivery have been seen.

Cerebral infarction may occur with cortical vein or sagittal sinus thrombosis in association with secondary tissue congestion after venous obstruction. Lateral sinus thrombosis may be associated with headache and a pseudotumor cerebri-like picture. Extension into the jugular may cause jugular foramen syndrome; variable cranial nerve palsies may be observed with cavernous sinus thrombosis.

Cerebral hemorrhages may be the presenting condition in sinus thrombosis. Imaging (MRI or CT) is generally diagnostic. The role of thrombophilic conditions is unclear. Prothrombotic conditions (protein C, protein S, or antithrombin deficiency), antiphospholipid syndrome, prothrombin G20210A mutation, and factor V Leiden can be important in DVT but, possibly, less determinant in this type of thrombosis.

The use of any anticoagulant must consider possible complications. During pregnancy, low-molecular-weight heparin (LMWH) in full anticoagulant doses should be continued throughout pregnancy, and LMWH or anticoagulants can be used for some 3 months postpartum. Acute CVT during pregnancy is generally managed with LMWH.

Compression of the iliac vein

The iliac artery in some patients and defined conditions may compress the left iliac vein. This may predispose to slower venous flow (particularly in some positions) and distal thrombosis of the left leg veins. The compression of the right vein is also possible but less common. Lordosis, in women, is an important cause accentuating the vein compression.

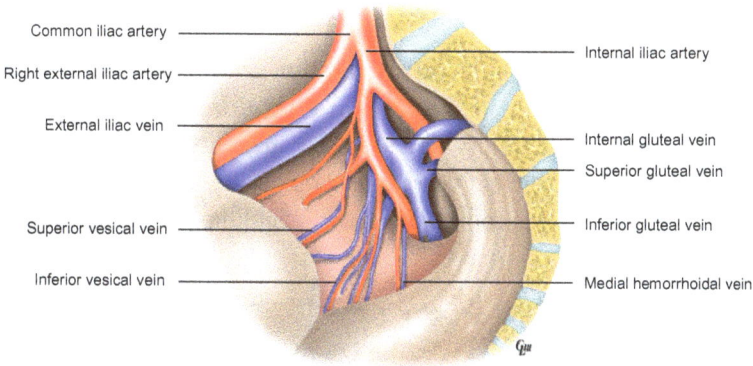

Angiological zebras

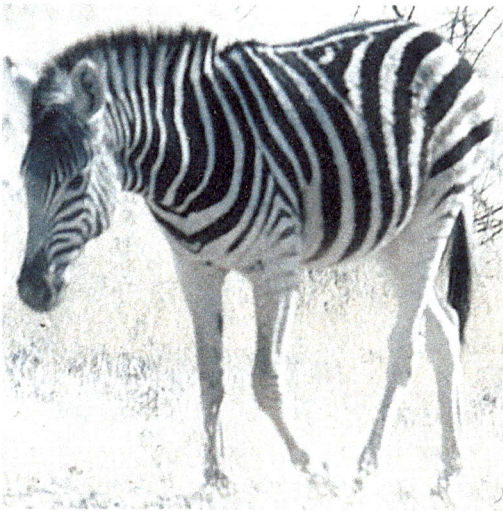

Some clinical problems are unusual and may be very dificult to diagnose and manage. In any "zebra", it is important to include in the diagnostic team a physician–vascular surgeon or circulation science specialist. Very often, the key of any difficult problem has a cardiovascular implication to be found.

Caval pseudothrombosis

A patient with massive bilateral obstruction arrives to our labs. After scans of the femoral, iliac and lower cava, no clot is found. Any thrombotic scan — for us (actually any scan, for any problem) — involves a visualization of the kidneys. A large tumor growing into the cava through a short right renal vein is found. The kidney and the pseudothrombus are subsequently excised.

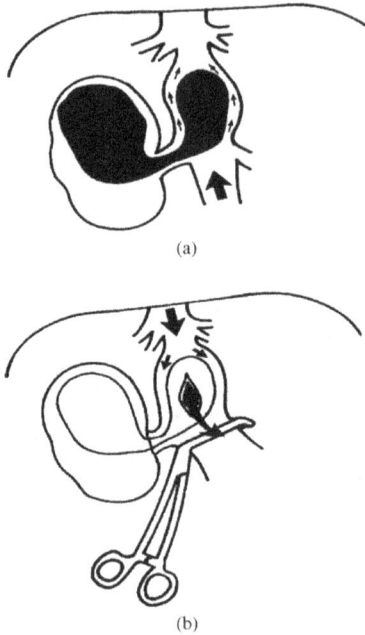

(a)

(b)

All the neoplastic lesions are below the liver levels. This type of pseudothrombus may reach the right atrium (some 15% of cases) being mostly retrohepatic (some 45% of cases). Caval surgery may produce a complete excision of the tumor. In some cases, a cardiopulmonary bypass is needed.

Splenic vein thrombosis

It may occur during an episode of pancreatitis, in subjects with pancreatic pseuodocysts, cysts or tumors and after trauma. In some patients, the diagnosis may be difficult with relatively limited symptoms. Splenomegaly is usually associated. Isolated splenic vein thrombosis may lead to variceal bleeding from the esophagus. In some cases, splenectomy is indicated. Splenic and portal hypertension may also be associated to this problem.

Unexplained edema and limb swelling

Thyroid problems may be associated to limb swelling. Pretibial edema was previously associated to hypothyroidism. However, different kinds of swelling are observed in many patients, particularly women with hidden thyroid conditions, particularly hypothyroidism.

Carotid screening considering the accessibility of the thyroid is now always associated to vascular screening. The incidence of thyroid problems also seems to be rising in connection with nuclear contaminations.

The Washingto

Mainly cloudy 66/48 • *Tomorrow: Shower 57/39* • **DETAILS, B10**   TUESDAY, OCTOBER 22, 2013

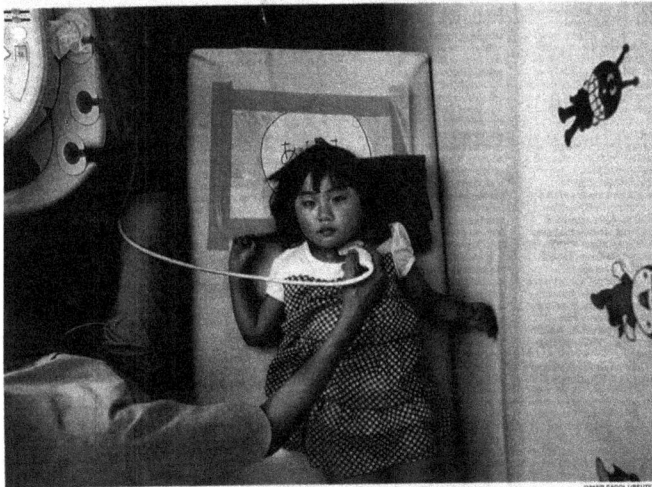

OMAR SAGOLL/REUTERS

A washout of a nuclear cleanup

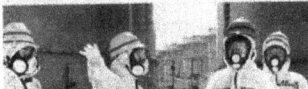

As Japan's crippled Fukushima plant struggles with buildup of toxic water, many blame operator

BY CHICO HARLAN
IN TOKYO

subsequently given a government bailout as its debts soared. The job of dismantling the facility was supposed to give Tepco an oppor-

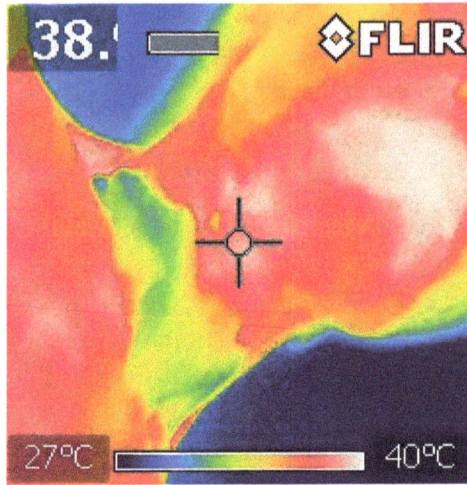

The FLIR scan above shows in seconds a thyroid at lower temperature (hypoactive) in a woman with unexplained leg swelling. The probe used to screen carotids is generally the same one used for thyroid scans. When scanning a carotid, it is useful to scan the thyroid at least for a preliminary evaluation. The evolution of many vascular conditions may be associated to thyroid malfunctions.

Thrombosis and travel: The LONFLIT studies

Prolonged air travel has been associated with deep venous thrombosis (DVT) and pulmonary embolism (PE). Prolonged bending and compression of leg veins (i.e., femoral, popliteal, soleal veins) on the edges of the seat could be a contributing factor to stasis and thrombosis. An increase in blood cell concentration, decreased fluid intake and the dry and low pressure environment in cabins have been implicated. Blood changes have been reported during simulated and real long flights, including fibrinogen and fibrinolysis alterations. Immobility, lower air pressure, and relative hypoxia may alter the spontaneous fibrinolytic activity and cause release of factors, leading to thrombosis.

Evidence suggests that there is a significant association between DVT and long flights. The prevalence of DVT is higher in predisposed, higher-risk subjects. Measures to prevent DVT include advice (changing positions, stretching, exercising, drinking, avoiding constrictive clothes). Subjects with risk factors for DVT, i.e., history of DVT, hormonal treatments, malignancy, recent surgery, should avoid if possible long flights and discuss protective measures with their physicians including postponing the flight. Effective preventive measures include elastic stockings and antithrombotic prophylaxis with LMWH or anticoagulants in very-high-risk conditions.

In the LONFLIT studies, the incidence of DVT in high-risk subjects was greater than 4%. The LONFLIT 2 study — prospective evaluation of DVT prevention with stockings — has shown that stockings decrease DVT incidence in long-haul flights. The LONFLIT 3 study has shown a reduction in DVT in high-risk subjects using LMWH. A specific product (Flite Tabs) including a combination of Pycnogenol and an oral profibrinolytic agent (NATTO) has also been useful to reduce edema and minor thrombotic events.

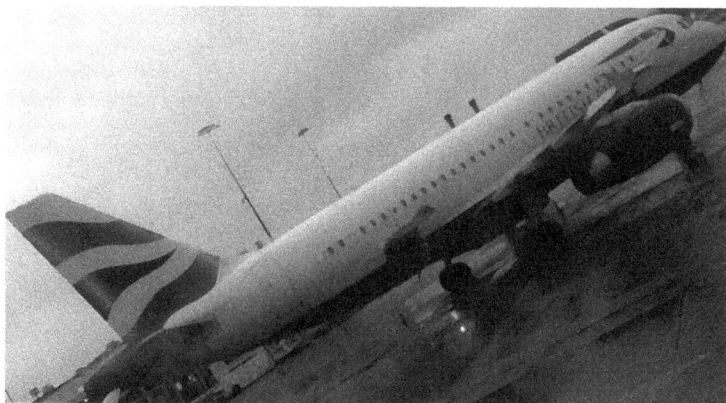

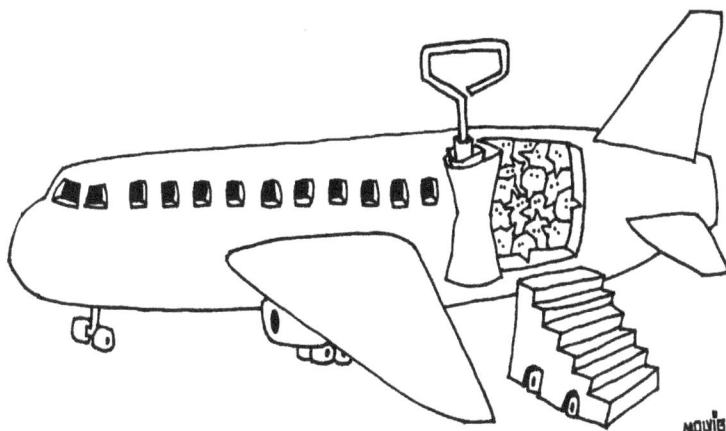

Forms

Form 1: DVT and/or deep venous incompetence.

Indicate level of obstruction or problem

Form 2: Superficical venous incompetence.

Date _____   Mr/Ms_____

Referring Doctor or Unit _____

Right leg   **Section (cm)**

Ant.   Post.

—11

—10

—9
—8
—7

—6

—5

—4

Left leg   —3
Ant.   Post.   —2
                                 —1

**Deep venous
system**   ☐ Cava
                          ☐ Iliacs
P = **Patency**   ☐ Common femoral
O = **Obstruction**   ☐ Superficial femoral
I = **Incompetence**   ☐ Popliteal
                          ☐ Posterior tibial
                          ☐ Distal veins

Duplex findings

\+ = **Reflux > 3 sec.**   _____

x = **Reflux < 3 sec.**   _____
                            _____

Note: "+"indicates significant reflux by Doppler or duplex (reflux longer than 3 s on standing). "×"indicates short lasting reflux (1–3 s).

Index

www.ingramcontent.com/pod-product-compliance
Lightning Source LLC
Chambersburg PA
CBHW050557190326

41458CB00007B/2081